Myofascial Pain and Dysfunction

Rolf Eichinger · Kerstin Klink

Myofascial Pain and Dysfunction

Diagnostics and Therapy

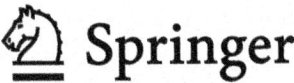 Springer

Rolf Eichinger
Hilpoltstein, Germany

Kerstin Klink
Roth, Germany

ISBN 978-3-662-68040-7   ISBN 978-3-662-68041-4   (eBook)
https://doi.org/10.1007/978-3-662-68041-4

Cover design: deblik Berlin

This Springer imprint is published by the registered company Springer-Verlag GmbH, DE, part of Springer Nature.
The registered company address is: Heidelberger Platz 3, 14197 Berlin, Germany

Preface

For years, I have been amazed at how many different complaints are triggered by disorders of the muscle/connective tissue apparatus, the "myofascial organ."

The symptoms of a disturbed myofascial apparatus are frequent and economically relevant. It would be all the more urgent to include knowledge about the diagnosis and therapy of myofascial disorders in the training of physicians.

This book provides an overview of pathomechanisms, symptoms, diagnostics, and therapy of myofascial disorders.

A particular focus is on manual therapy methods, which are discussed in more detail in the second part of the book.

These are explained using the KLINEA method, which also shows quickly learnable diagnostic and therapeutic options for the physician.

Hilpoltstein   Dr. Rolf Eichinger
Roth   Kerstin Klink
in the summer of 2019

Contents

List of Figures

About the Authors

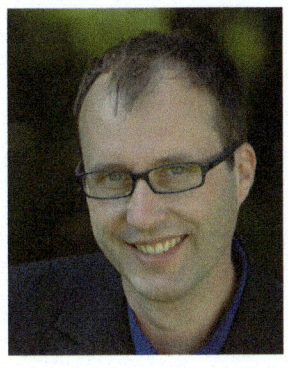

Dr. Rolf Eichinger since 7/2002 own general practice (chirotherapy, nutritional medicine, diving medicine, emergency medicine)

5/1999–4/2002 Assistant physician in the general practice Auhof/Hilpoltstein

3/1997–4/1999 Assistant physician at Hersbruck Hospital (Internal Medicine, Gynecology, and Surgery)

10/1997 Dissertation on the filtration performance of the nose (ENT Clinic Erlangen)

3/1993–10/1993 Tropical medicine at Bukoba/Tanzania Hospital

3/1990–10/1996 Medical studies at the Friedrich-Alexander University Erlangen

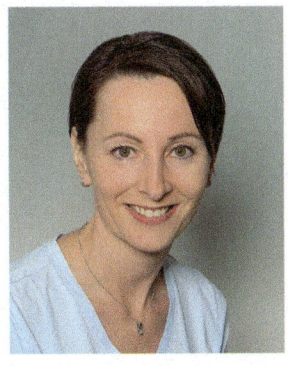

Kerstin Klink since 07/2003 own physiotherapy practice

01/2000–05/2003 freelance work

10/1997–07/1999 Training as a manual therapist

10/1997–12/1999 Median Rehabilitation Center Ansbach

07/1997–10/1997 Internship at Edenreha/Regenstauf

10/1994–07/1997 Training as a state-recognized physiotherapist in Bad Abbach

Introduction

1

When I switched to the outpatient area of general medicine after my clinical training in 1998, I was very surprised by the discrepancy between the patient collective of the clinic and the cases of a general practitioner's practice. This is probably the case for every newcomer. While in the hospital, more severe internal medical conditions were treated, in everyday practice, 80% of the cases encountered are functional diseases. Dysfunctions, which initially cannot be assigned to a clearly defined disease, such as those learned in the study. This phenomenon can certainly be extended to the entire outpatient area. Organ specialists face similar problems when they come from the clinic.

Thus, not every prolonged diarrhea has to have ulcerative colitis or Crohn's disease as its cause. The diagnosis here is usually irritable bowel syndrome, which does not lead to any rational treatment and does not help anyone. The situation is similar with the diseases of all other specialist areas, especially those from surgery and orthopedics.

In my file, there are about 10,000 patients, of whom about 1300 appear quarterly in the consultation. Due to the range of services offered by the practice, I mainly have younger patients (Fig. 1.1).

The largest proportion of my patients come to my consultation because of unclear pain and other functional, i.e., non-somatic structural problems. These very diverse symptoms affect all possible regions, take on various forms, and are very volatile in their localization.

Unlike what is learned in studies and clinics, about 80% of these functional syndromes are neither traumatic nor skeletal in origin. The often-assumed disc damage or even prolapse causes much fewer complaints than expected. I think that many patients over 50 have spondylarthrosis, disc protrusions, and even sequesters that are absolutely painless.

In his dissertation, Torsten Pippig examined spinal MRIs of 488 symptom-free men aged 17–24 in 2008. Here is a brief excerpt from the work:

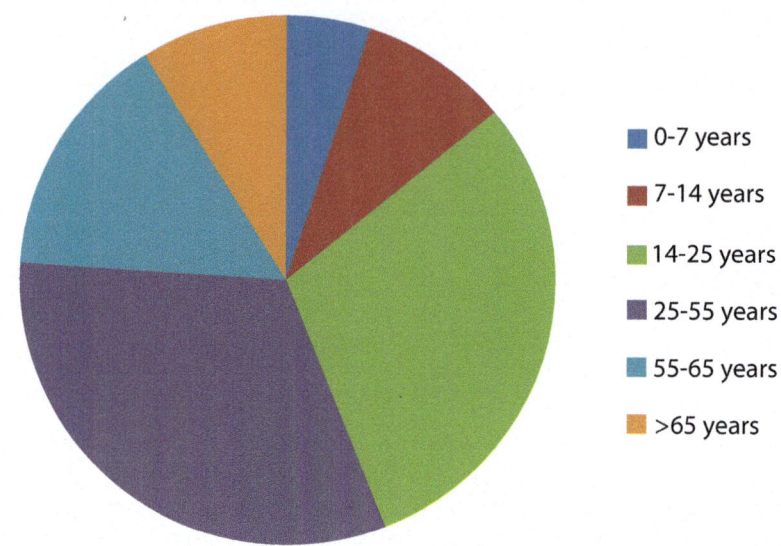

Fig. 1.1 Age distribution of the patients in my practice

"[…] in 81.2% (396), noticeable or abnormal changes in the spine and spinal cord were seen: 15 spondylolyses/spondylolistheses (3.1%), 51 lumbosacral transitional vertebrae (10.4%), 5 block vertebrae (1.0%), 1 butterfly vertebra, 25 spines (5.1%) with a total of 38 vertebral body hemangiomas, 158 spines (32.4%) showed Scheuermann's changes, and 23 spines (4.7%) showed spinal cord changes (21 hydromyelia, 2 sacral Tarlov cysts, and 1 sacral ectasia). In addition, asymptomatic disc changes were seen in 239 of the applicants (49.0%). A total of 29 disc herniations were described in 26 asymptomatic applicants."[1]

And these were young people!

Actually, one can neither do anything with all the circulating "diagnoses" for said syndromes, nor do any meaningful therapies derive from the obscure models. What is an ischialgia, a pinched nerve, a "jumped out" vertebra, a nerve inflammation, and all the other strange causes of pain cited in the common literature? In the general medicine guidelines available to me, there is absolutely nothing about myogeloses or blockage complaints, although they are very common. Unrecognized, they lead to nonsensical diagnostics and result in unsuccessful therapies.

Common views on the cause of pain, dizziness, or other felt sensations usually lead to NSAID or corticoid therapies, because in the opinion of many colleagues, there must always be inflammation behind "Dolor." Unfortunately, most forget over the years that inflammation also includes Rubor and Calor, which are

---

[1] On the frequency of asymptomatic spinal and spinal cord changes in young men - an MRI study of 488 symptom-free men between 17 and 24 years, T. Pippig 2008.

practically never found in atraumatic, non-infectious pain conditions. It is therefore not surprising that anti-inflammatory therapy approaches do very little, often even causing harm.

Therefore, based on my 30-year experience as a chiropractor and after 20 years in general medicine, I am trying to present a theory on myofascial syndromes here. My co-author Kerstin Klink, a physiotherapist who has been in her own practice for 20 years, presents the physiotherapeutic treatment approaches in the second part of this book. In doing so, she combines the relevant, essential techniques of many different physiotherapeutic currents and schools of thought in the method called "KLINEA." This way, much "ballast" that has little significance in everyday clinical practice is omitted.

The second part of this book is intended to inform the physician about the possibilities and indications of physiotherapy, as close cooperation and mutual understanding of each other's actions are often lacking but important. Coordinated collaboration between medical and physiotherapy practices saves a lot of unnecessary diagnostics, pointless drug therapies, and thus conserves resources.

Much of the model of myogelotic syndromes presented here is hypothetical but corresponds to our observations and therapeutic successes.

We would very much like to see a future scientific investigation of our hypotheses in order to finally expand knowledge about one of the most common health disorders and incorporate it into the training of doctors and physiotherapists.

Myofascial Trigger Points or Blockages

2

Contents

The analysis of my practice data shows that approximately 70% of practice visits are due to myofascial adhesions or blockages with various symptoms.

Only 14% of contacts occur due to traumas of any kind.

56% of patients come to the consultation due to pain as a result of local disturbances of muscles and fascia. In my practice, this amounts to about 750 patients per quarter!

The functional unit of muscles and connective tissue represents its own, the so-called "myofascial organ". Said disturbances of the myofascial organ manifest as tensions or tissue swellings. I would like to refer to these swellings as myofascial adhesions or blockages, which on the one hand show a "congested", subedematous tissue structure, which is either actively painful or reacts painfully to manipulation.

The example of a young cat, in which all tissue layers are soft and elastically displaceable and in which no pain is triggered when properly "cuddled", helps students. In the case of myogeloses, the tissue is not, as in the aforementioned cat, elastic, soft, and displaceable, but appears stuck together, hardened, swollen.

2.1   Finding Criteria of Myofascial Adhesion = Blockage

- Swollen tissue
- Stuck together tissue layers, mobility of skin, subcutaneous fat tissue, myom and fascial compartments is reduced or abolished

- Pain triggering already by gentle manipulation of the tissue
- Chain-like course (see Fascial Chains)

The diagnosis of a myofascial adhesion is therefore clinical and can only be achieved through the manual examination of the patient. So, one must touch the patient. Often, just the touches during a greeting, such as placing a hand on the shoulder, etc., are enough to get an impression of the extent of the patient's blockages.

2.2   Common Symptoms of Blockages

- Tension headaches
- Migraine/Fibromyalgia (?)
- Visual disturbances, especially Mouches voilantes
- Vertigo
- Tinnitus
- Sudden hearing loss
- Dysphagia, feeling of a lump in the throat
- Insertion tendopathies (tennis elbow)
- Arthralgia, sometimes with inflammatory effusions
- Muscle pain
- Thoracic sensations with symptoms of a heart attack
- Upper abdominal pressure sensations often with nausea
- Groin pain
- Back pain
- Painful restrictions of movement
- Tendovaginitis

It is a myth that extreme blood pressure causes headaches, dizziness, or sudden hearing loss. At least, I have never experienced it in 20 years of emergency medical service. Patients usually have blockage-related symptoms, then become anxious and reactively develop high blood pressure. Patients with myogeloses always appear relatively healthy, which is not the case with headaches caused by a subarachnoid hemorrhage or thoracic pain caused by coronary heart disease.

Of course, it is up to personal experience and extended diagnostics to distinguish harmless blockages from serious illnesses. Fortunately, the latter are much rarer. I estimate that 80% of my emergency medical service calls were triggered by myofascial disorders and actually required a chiropractor, physiotherapist, or other manual therapist instead of an emergency doctor. As an emergency doctor, I have often unblocked patients, which usually worked, and I never had to return to a patient because a serious disorder was present after all. Only once did I have a 32-year-old truck driver who had thoracic pain at 7 a.m. His ECG was inconspicuous. In the hospital, however, an NSTEMI was revealed. This was the only case in all those years where coronary heart disease was hiding behind the suspected myogelosis.

Myofascial disorders are so common that all cultures have developed massage, gymnastics, and manipulation techniques for treatment. Just think of Shiatsu massage, yoga, acupuncture, neural therapy, manual therapy, osteopathy, Thai massages, or chiropractic, which has its origins in the indigenous cultures of North America.

I myself learned chiropractic, among other things, from a teacher who was taught it in Russian captivity by a Siberian doctor of the Red Army to whom he was assigned.

All these therapy forms identify disorders by palpating tissue swellings (e.g., Kibler's fold) or painful muscle tension, which are then directly massaged or otherwise manipulated. The insertion of an acupuncture needle or the injection of a local anesthetic is ultimately a neuromanipulative measure, as are manual procedures.

Every therapist notices that myofascial disorders often run in chains. That, for example, the classic tennis elbow always goes hand in hand with a disturbed fascial blockage chain over the deltoid muscle, trapezius muscle, and into the neck muscles, and actually usually originates from the proximal disturbances.

Pathophysiology

3

Contents

Even during my studies as a newcomer to chiropractic, I found it striking that back, neck, shoulder arm pain, etc. often improved significantly or even disappeared completely immediately after manipulation of the involved segments or areas.

So it cannot be inflammatory processes, as these subside but do not disappear. The same applies to traumatic symptoms. Therefore, with blockages, heat is always more helpful than cold, which would reduce inflammatory complaints.

Myofascial geloses (= blockage) must therefore be of neurological origin. The cause is a misregulation of muscle tension, connective tissue metabolism, and vegetative regulation, which arises or is mediated centrally.

This is consistent with the observation that a disturbance can cause blockages that often occur at completely different locations than the triggering disturbance.

I once treated a chimney sweep who had persistent Achilles tendon pain with tendinosis, which incapacitated him for almost a year and remained therapy-resistant despite cortisone injections, NRSA, and other orthopedic treatment attempts. I suspected a dental focus as the trigger, but an OPG (odontopantomogram) and an NMR showed no pathological findings in this area. Only a thermography showed a significant increase in temperature at a tooth without any clinical symptoms. Upon opening the tooth, a lot of pus was released, the tooth was extracted, and the Achilles tendon pain disappeared after just one week.

Since we still know far too little about our brain to develop conclusive, neuroanatomical-functional models of myofascial disorders, only a black-box model remains as a solution.

The central nervous system subsumes all functions of our organism into a whole. Sensory-tactile, perceptive, proprioceptive, vegetative, emotional, psychological, etc. information is measured, analyzed, compared, stored, and triggers reactions in an integrative manner. Thus, there are thousands of control loops that all need to be integrated and calculated together to enable adequate control of the organism itself in interaction with its environment.

I find the idea of a huge computer network helpful in this context, in which, despite all its genius, control disorders also occur. That is, with completely intact "hardware," there are still "software problems" that result in functional disorders in an organism. With complete structural health, there is still pain, limited mobility, and other functional symptoms, such as bladder emptying disorders, diarrhea, or visual disturbances, among many others (Fig. 3.1).

If there are incorrect information or pathologies that interfere with the calculation of afferent signals, this results in incorrect counter-control in the efferences.

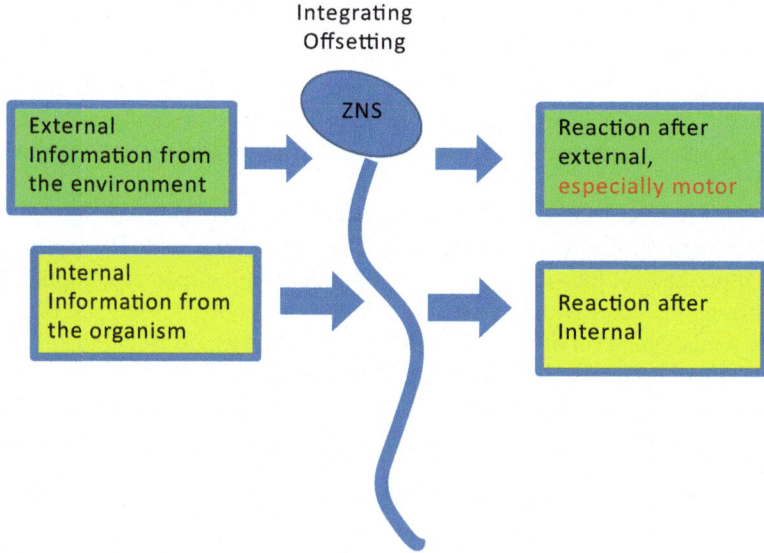

Fig. 3.1 Simple model of organism control

A simple example is the discrepancy between position sense information and visual impression on a ship. From the inner ear comes the information that the organism is swaying, which does not correspond to the visual impression of an unmoving environment. Our CNS initially cannot cope with this situation, especially if it has no prior experience with said condition. It then causes massive nausea and feelings of weakness in many people, often forcing them to rest and close their eyes, which then improves the situation. There is a massive gastrointestinal symptomatology with complete health of the gastrointestinal tract.

Another common example is the "draft". Patients come with torticollis and extreme cervical tension because they fell asleep, for example, at the open window of a car. They then say they caught a "draft". Apparently, a uniform sensory input leads to a disturbance in the processing in the central nervous system, which then causes blockages with massive myofascial tension. Certainly, there is no trauma caused by the wind.

The same mechanism is used by the Chinese water drop torture, in which a victim is dripped with a water drop at the same frequency on the head. The tortured person develops massive myofascial pain in a short time.

I believe that any monotonous neurological input leads to malfunctions of our organism, which result in blockages.

This is also shown by the frequency of these complaints in endurance athletes.

Road cyclists, who always remain in the same position and movement, are much more affected by blockage complaints than mountain bikers, who constantly vary their movement and posture. The same applies to joggers who run on asphalt versus those who have to vary their movements on a forest track. The typical forearm tendovaginitis after monotonous work is not an "overload", but a misdirection of the synovial supply of the tendon sheath due to blockages and a disturbed relaxation of the arm muscles (see "Lot passage"). Monotony in movement is, in my opinion, also the cause of complaints in office workers.

The cause of a myofascial gelosis is therefore a neurological misdirection, which manifests itself in the myofascial organ. At the very center of the events are our muscles and connective tissue.

A lot has changed scientifically in the last ten years.

Connective tissue connects and separates organ and muscle compartments, it connects them together like the cables of a suspension bridge, integrates the skeleton, and serves as a storage for all "lines" of an organism, such as blood and lymph vessels, nerve pathways, and interstitial, humoral elements, such as mediators and immune cells. It is influenced by all processes of this organism and forms a unity with all parts of it (Fig. 3.2).

Connective tissue, like any organ, is innervated afferently and efferently and can mediate pain.

It has its own smooth muscle fibers that modulate connective tissue tension, and afferent mechano- and thermosensitive as well as polymodal nociceptors,

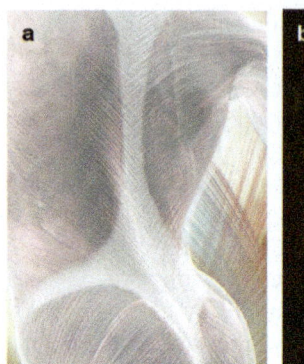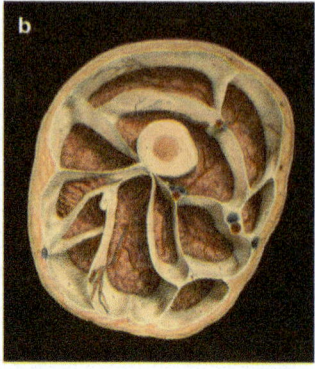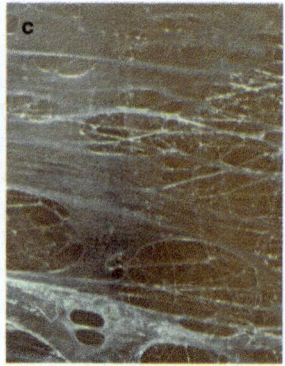

Fig. 3.2 The fascial system includes large aponeuroses, such as the first layer of the thoracolumbar fascia (**a**), but it also defines the compartments of the skeletal musculature (**b**) and all organs. The internal connective tissue structure consists of a collagen framework, which is embedded in a semi-liquid, gel-like basic substance (**c**). (From British Journal of Sportsmed. *Fascial tissue research in sports medicine: from molecules to tissue adaptation, injury and diagnostics: consensus statement* Martina Zügel et al. 2018)

which are in turn controlled by efferents[1] . Still misunderstood receptor systems, such as calcitonin gene-related peptide (CGRP) receptors or substance P receptors, are involved in myofascial pain syndromes. Contractions of the muscle fibers of the myofascial organ under the influence of stress hormones have also been demonstrated[2]

I could imagine that even the semi-liquid matrix in which collagen fibers "swim" changes its viscosity in a controlled manner, similar to dilatant colloidal dispersions, as used in shock absorbers.

The myofascial organ contains Pacini and Ruffini-corpuscles as well as Golgi tendon organs, which measure vibrations, pressure, acceleration, and tissue tension.

Robert Schleip (Univ. Ulm), who has made a significant contribution to fascia research, refers to connective tissue as the largest sensory organ of the so-called "sixth sense," the sensory organ of proprioception.[3]

In the holistic unity of an organism, the connective tissue, like the myofascial organ itself, is connected to everything and influenced by everything. Fig. 3.3 shows direct influencing factors that trigger effects on connective tissue.

The myofascial organ is involved in every movement, whether voluntary or involuntary, it stores kinetic energy, which it can also release again, like a bow with its string.

---

[1] Tesarz 2009.

[2] Schleip 2015.

[3] Schleip 2003.

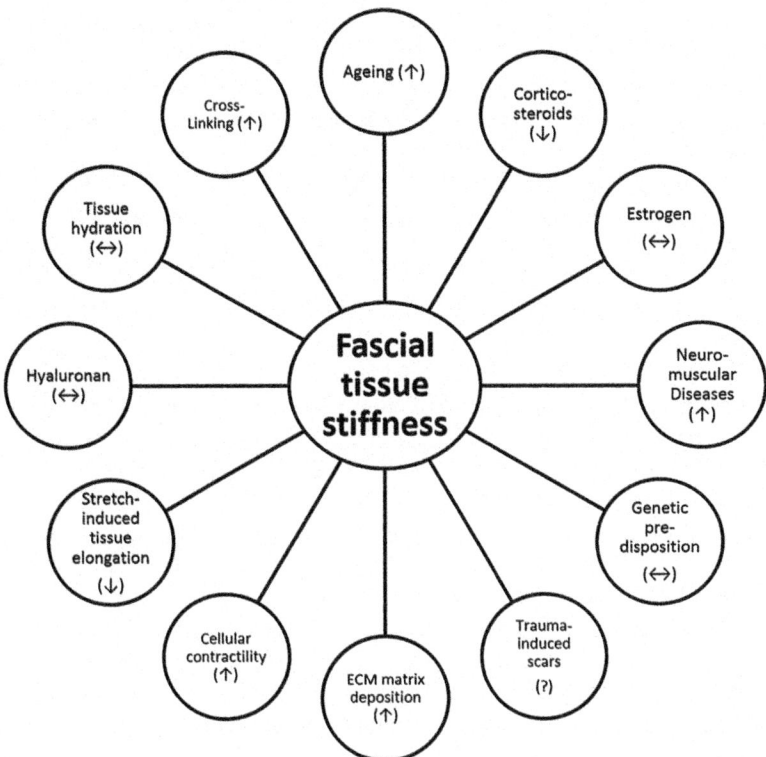

Fig. 3.3 Influencing factors on connective tissue consistency (connective tissue stiffness). (From British Journal of Sportsmed. *Fascial tissue research in sports medicine: from molecules to tissue adaptation, injury and diagnostics: consensus statement* Martina Zügel et al.)

Since the myofascial organ has the task of dynamically aligning our body in space, it integrates countless force vectors that act simultaneously on the body. In daily treatment practice, it has proven useful to distinguish between compressed and extended compartments. It is noticeable that pain usually occurs in the extended areas, which can be treated through therapy on the compressed antagonist. More on this later.

The myofascial organ is holistically networked with all parts of the body. Therefore, a disturbance of the myofascial organ can manifest itself in a variety of symptoms.

3.1 Myofascial Knots

As already described, the myofascial organ forms a unity with all parts of our body.

However, some areas are particularly complex and therefore more susceptible to disturbances due to anatomical and neurological conditions. One day it became clear to me that blockages are usually found in identical areas.

I refer to these areas as knots, in reference to their use in statics. Knots are places of tension transmission, or connections or redirection of different tension vectors. As seen in bridge constructions or the rigging of a ship with masts, shrouds, spreaders, and stays.

Force vectors project into the three-dimensional structure of the knots. In the knots, these dynamic force vectors are integrated, neutralized, redirected, or amplified to ensure the correct alignment and movement of our body in an energy-saving and efficient manner.

Interestingly, these knots are always located at arch structures, which can best absorb and redirect tension vectors. In addition, all proximal knots contain important arch structures in the horizontal plane, which are extremely important for therapy and are therefore mentioned below in the list following the designation of the knots.

From a neurological point of view, knots are exposed because a particularly large amount of information enters the CNS here, is partially processed at the segmental level, and results in efferent signals. Motor and vegetative efferences are concentratedly connected in them. Just consider that walking movements are generated at the sacral level and are only modified by higher CNS levels. Therefore, it is not surprising that blockages are mainly found at knots. Where a lot of calculations have to be made, errors also occur more frequently.

I have defined the following knots for my daily work:

1. Calvarial accounts   Calvaria, skull base
2. Pharyngeal node   Palate/oral floor
3. Upper thoracic node   Pleural domes
4. Lower thoracic node   Diaphragm
5. Sacral node   Pelvic floor
6. Elbow node
7. Carpal node
8. Knee node
9. Foot node

Where 1. to 5. form the group of proximal nodes and 6. to 9. the distal nodes. The proximal nodes are much more important here, as most disturbances originate from here, which then also cause disturbances in the peripheral nodes.

Among the proximal nodes, the pharyngeal node occupies a key position. Pathologies have a particularly strong effect on the myofascial apparatus here, probably due to the concentrated and demanded computing power of our CNS. The area of this node accounts for about 30% of the sensory and motor computing power of our cortex, as shown in Fig. 3.4.

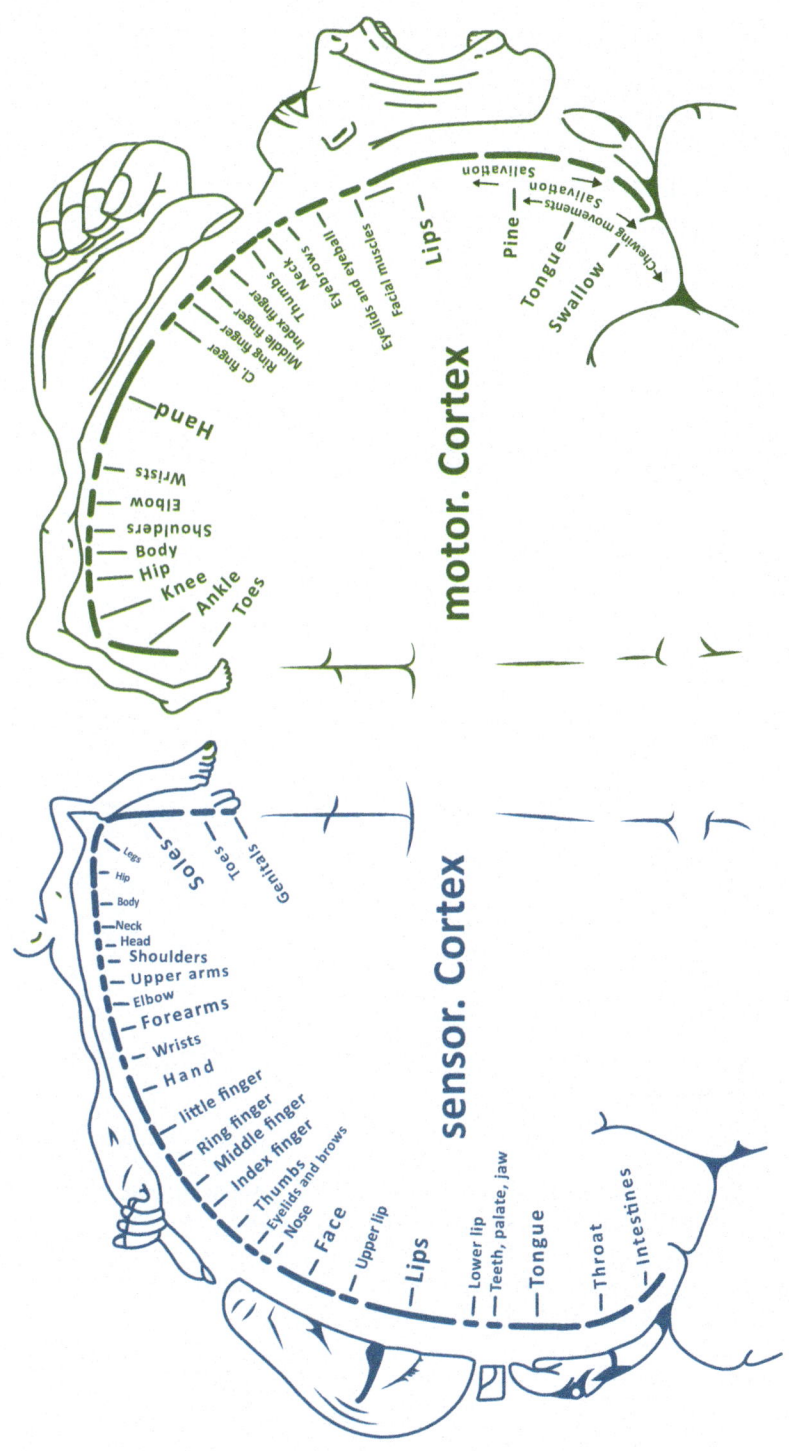

Fig. 3.4 Humunculus

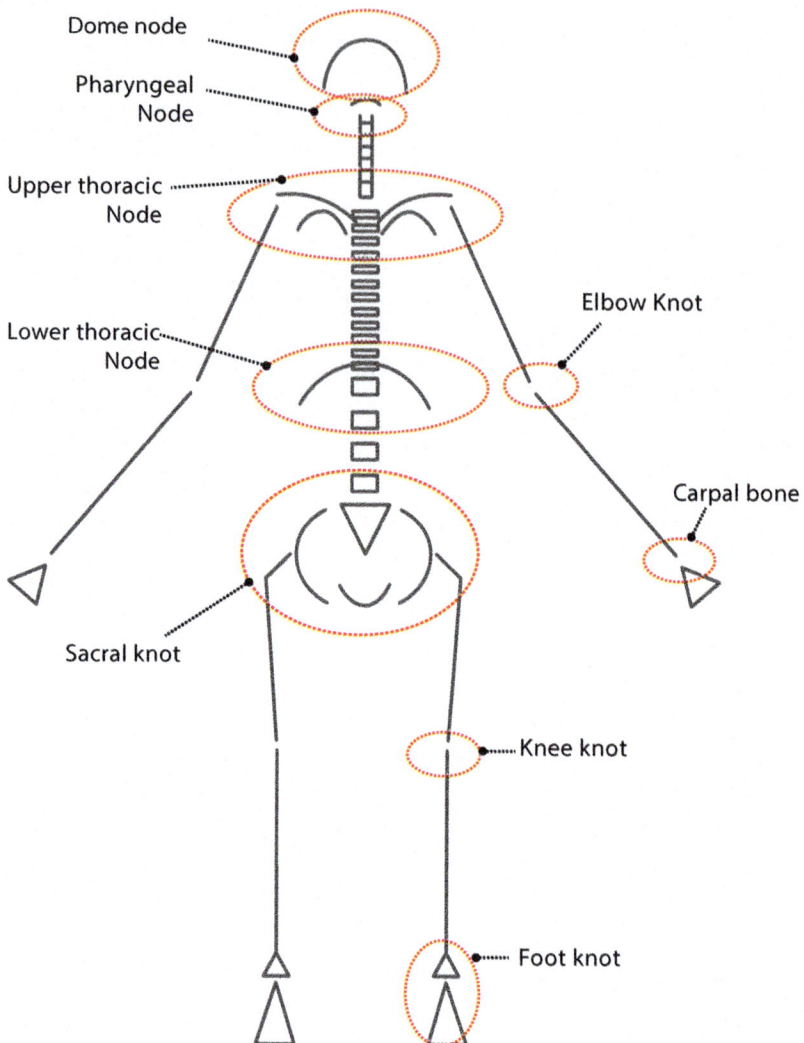

Dome node

Pharyngeal Node

Upper thoracic Node

Lower thoracic Node

Elbow Knot

Carpal bone

Sacral knot

Knee knot

Foot knot

Fig. 3.5 Myofascial nodes

Of course, countless more nodes could be defined, but I would like to present a simple, proven tool and model for daily therapy with patients (Fig. 3.5).

Nodes actually only summarize all functions of the respective region. In the following, the region of the node with the most important anatomical structures, joints, afferents, and functions involved is described. The definition is a clinical-functional one. All nodes are closely functionally coupled and represent key regions of tension absorption and distribution of vectorial forces of the myofascial apparatus.

Since the myofascial organ primarily fulfills mechanical tasks in the context of the organism's movements, it is always particularly affected by sclerosing organ diseases that reduce the mobility, glideability, and elasticity of organs. Liver cirrhosis disturbs more than gallbladder concrements, lung fibrosis more than asthma, meteorism more than a colon tumor, pericardial effusions more than coronary heart disease, kidney cysts more than glomerulitis, etc.

3.1.1 Calotte Bode (= KK)

Region
Skull cap, orbital region, small neck muscles, M. frontalis, M. temporalis, eye muscles.

Afferents/Efferents
Visual and sensorimotor information of the region.

Functions
Psychomotor, oculomotor, sense of sight.

Common pathological effectors in the node area
Visual impairments, strabismus, angle anomalies, scars.

Common symptoms
Tension headaches, migraine, visual sensations such as Mouches volantes, ptosis.

3.1.2 Pharyngeal Node (= PK)

Region
Hard and soft palate with small and large chewing muscles, tongue, pharyngeal muscles, M. sternocleidomastoideus, M. digastricus, M. omohyoideus, platysma, Eustachian tube, ear, paranasal sinuses, pharynx, jaw, upper cervical spine.

Afferents/Efferents
Taste, hearing, balance, sense of smell, sensorimotor information of the region (partly from the hands), cervical ganglion sup.

Functions
Motor function of the cranio-cervical junction, speaking, swallowing, chewing, tasting, smelling, hearing, psychomotor, integration of head position.

Common pathological effectors in the node area
Psychological stress, bruxism, sinusitis (including allergic), cerumen, dental foci, scars (thyroid resections).

Common symptoms
Vertigo, hypacusis (sudden hearing loss), tinnitus, temporomandibular joint pain, functional eustachian tube dysfunction, muscular otalgia, dysphagia, globus sensation.

3.1.3   Upper Thoracic Node (= OTK)

Region
Lower cervical spine, upper thoracic spine up to approx. Th3, shoulder joint, pleural domes, sternoclavicular joint, M. trapezius, all shoulder muscles, shoulder joint.

Afferents/Efferents
Sensomotor information of the region (partly from the hands), Ganglion cervic. med., Ganglion stellatum.

Functions
Shoulder-/Arm-/Hand-Mobility.

Common pathological effectors in the node area
Tension vectors from the pharyngeal node, which are intercepted and redirected here, scars (thyroid resections), compliance-reducing lung diseases, pericarditis, hypertrophic heart diseases, coronary heart disease.

Common symptoms
Shoulder pain, frozen shoulder, limited mobility of the cervical spine, neck pain, thoracic pain, thoracic feelings of constriction, tendovaginitis in the arms, insertion tendopathies in the arms (tennis elbow), paresthesias of the hands, finger joint arthralgias, nocturnal lymphatic congestion with finger swelling.

3.1.4   Lower Thoracic Node (= UTK)

Region
Lower thoracic spine, upper lumbar spine, renal fascia, diaphragm, liver, stomach, pancreas, kidneys, spleen, transverse colon, heart.

Afferents/Efferents
Sensomotor information from the region, sympathetic nervous system with Ganglion coeliacum/mesentericum sup.

Functions
Motor function of the thoracolumbar transition, abdominal breathing, digestion with the functions of the upper abdominal organs.

Common pathological effectors in the node area
Gastritis, meteorism, irritable bowel syndrome, colitis, liver diseases (especially sclerosing), irritative cough, pericarditis, hypertrophic heart diseases.

Common symptoms
Thoracic pain, thoracic feelings of constriction, breathing difficulties, epigastric pressure sensations, nausea, heart sensations without somatic correlate.

3.1.5 Sacral Node (= SN)

Region
Lower lumbar spine, sacrum, lumbar aponeurosis, gluteal muscles, small pelvic muscles (obturator, piriformis, etc.), lumbar muscles, inferior hypogastric ganglion, sensorimotor from the region, iliopsoas muscle, groin, bladder, uterus, ovaries, prostate, pelvic floor, rectum, urethra, vagina.

Afferents/Efferents
Sensorimotor from the region and from the legs/feet, inferior mesenteric ganglion, superior hypogastric plexus, sacral parasympathetic, motor autonomous spinal centers.

Functions
Motor function of lower lumbar spine/pelvis/legs, parasympathetic control of the intestine from the left colic flexure, defecation, micturition, sexual functions.

Common pathological effectors in the node area
Meteorism, uterine fibroids, ovarian cysts, cesarean section scars, pelvic adhesions, prostate hyperplasia, helminthiasis especially in children, pelvic congestion syndrome (15% of all women >40 years).

Common Symptoms
Lumboischialgia, bladder emptying disorders, groin pain, insertion tendopathies in the legs (up to knee joint effusions), Achilles tendon pain, "heel spur" = myogelosis of the plantar aponeurosis.
The following are the peripheral nodes, which have a more mechanical significance and therefore also show more mechanical symptoms. The periphery has few pathological effectors, apart from obvious traumas and foot arch disorders. I will therefore only list the region and typical symptoms here.

3.1.6 Elbow Node (= EN)

Region
Elbow joint with adjacent muscle groups.

Common Symptoms
Insertion tendopathies (tennis elbow), limited range of motion.

3.1.7   Carpal Node (= CN)

Region
Radio-ulnar-carpal joint, carpal joints, entire hand with all muscles in this region.

Common Symptoms
Limited range of motion.

3.1.8   Knee Node (= KnN)

Region
Knee region.

Common Symptoms
Knee pain, sometimes with reactive effusions.

3.1.9   Foot Node (= FN)

Region
Ankle joints and foot with all muscles.

Common pathological effectors in the node area
Scar disorders and foot arch disorders.

Common Symptoms
Limited range of motion and pain.

3.2   Fascial Chains

Every therapist notices that painful blockages are never isolated locally, but always occur in chains. For example, with a painful shoulder, there is always a connection to the pharyngeal node via the M. sternocleidomastoideus, the M. omohyoideus, the neck muscles, or the laryngeal suspension and their associated fasciae.

Of course, the entire skeleton is always tense in its small segmental compartments at every anatomical level. However, clinically, the large tension chains are much more important because they cause most of the symptoms at the nodes or are activated by pathologies in the node—thus entering a pathological tension.

These large force vector arcs, which always cross frontally or sagittally, span the entire skeleton and dynamically stabilize it, are referred to as fascial chains.

Figures 3.7 and 3.8 show a schematic representation of the fascial chains, with all chains being symmetrical. For better clarity, however, they are only shown on one side of the body.

All fascial chains (FK) run over the nodes in the frontal and sagittal planes.

In these planes, they tense the skeleton triangularly (as in a building or the rigging of a sailing ship), so that all force vectors are stabilized in the plane. Movement is then only possible if the chains are coordinatedly lengthened or shortened.

I divide fascial chains into unilateral and crossing, with the latter not necessarily crossing, but often running obliquely, so that they are again triangularly tense with each other.

Fascial chains stabilize the dynamics and elastically catch them at the end of a movement, storing kinetic energy and releasing it, often redirected, for the next movement.

My co-author, Kerstin Klink, has developed her own physiotherapeutic technique (KLINEA), which is briefly described in the second part of this book. In this technique, the term "plumb" plays an important role. We understand it as a state of balanced relaxation. "Being in plumb" does not mean to relax motionlessly, but rather, every organism in motion must repeatedly pass through the plumb state to briefly relax and, from this moment, move into the next movement. Plumb states can also exist simultaneously alongside tension states. For example, a cyclist, when pedaling with one leg, must briefly come into plumb with the other leg to avoid tension. Sacral, knee, and foot nodes must briefly relax in the suspension of their fascial chain in the plumb to allow a regenerative phase in the movement. After passing through the plumb, one side then switches to power output, and the opposite side experiences the plumb passage. This perpetual alternation between dynamics and plumb passage is absolutely necessary for maintaining health under mechanical stress. Inexperienced athletes who are not yet skilled in their technique often practice their sport without plumb passages. If tennis players or swimmers remain "cramped," they develop typical fascial disorders, such as tennis elbow or neck problems (Fig. 3.6).

With some practice, it is very easy to feel which chains are pathologically tense or, more precisely, where myogeloses, i.e., reduced elasticity, exist.

In my daily practice, I describe pathologically activated chains according to their course.

For example:
Left gonalgia with blockade of the right temporomandibular joint (e.g., in bruxism) with lateral FK crossing from OTK to UTK, left rib arch traction-sensitive, activated FK lateral left over SK with activation of the M. tensor fasciae latae.
  or also
Lumbago L2-L4 in meteorism with activation of the lateral and crossing FK, UTK to SK (Figs. 3.7 and 3.8).

Fig. 3.6 Tensioning force vectors that are triangularly "knotted" together, thus stabilizing the body in space. These triangular pulls can be seen in every aponeurosis (see Fig. 3.2a)

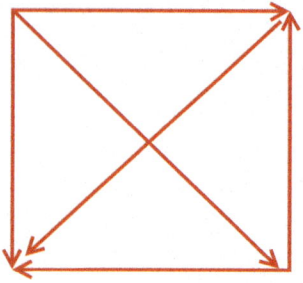

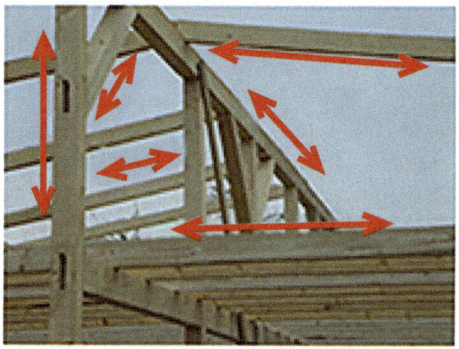

Since this work is aimed at the professional therapist who is well acquainted with anatomy and neurology, I will not name all the muscles or myofascial parts of a chain.

Chapter summary: Causes of myofascial syndromes, statistics from practice.

3.3   Causes of Myofascial Syndromes

In my opinion, the trigger for myogeloses of the myofascial organ lies either in consistency-changing pathologies that disturb the motor dynamics of the entire organism or in the direct affection of neurological processes.

Particularly disruptive are changes in compliance of organs, i.e., changes in the consistency of the organ structure. The reduced ability of an organ to follow general body movements due to loss of elasticity leads, on the one hand, directly to disturbances in the tone of the myofascial organ with direct activation of nociceptors. On the other hand, there are neurological misregulations because the central nervous integration of the general body sensation, with position information, movement planning, and movement control is disturbed. As a result, the interplay of tension and relaxation of the myofascial organ is no longer balanced, which in turn triggers the activation of nociceptors.

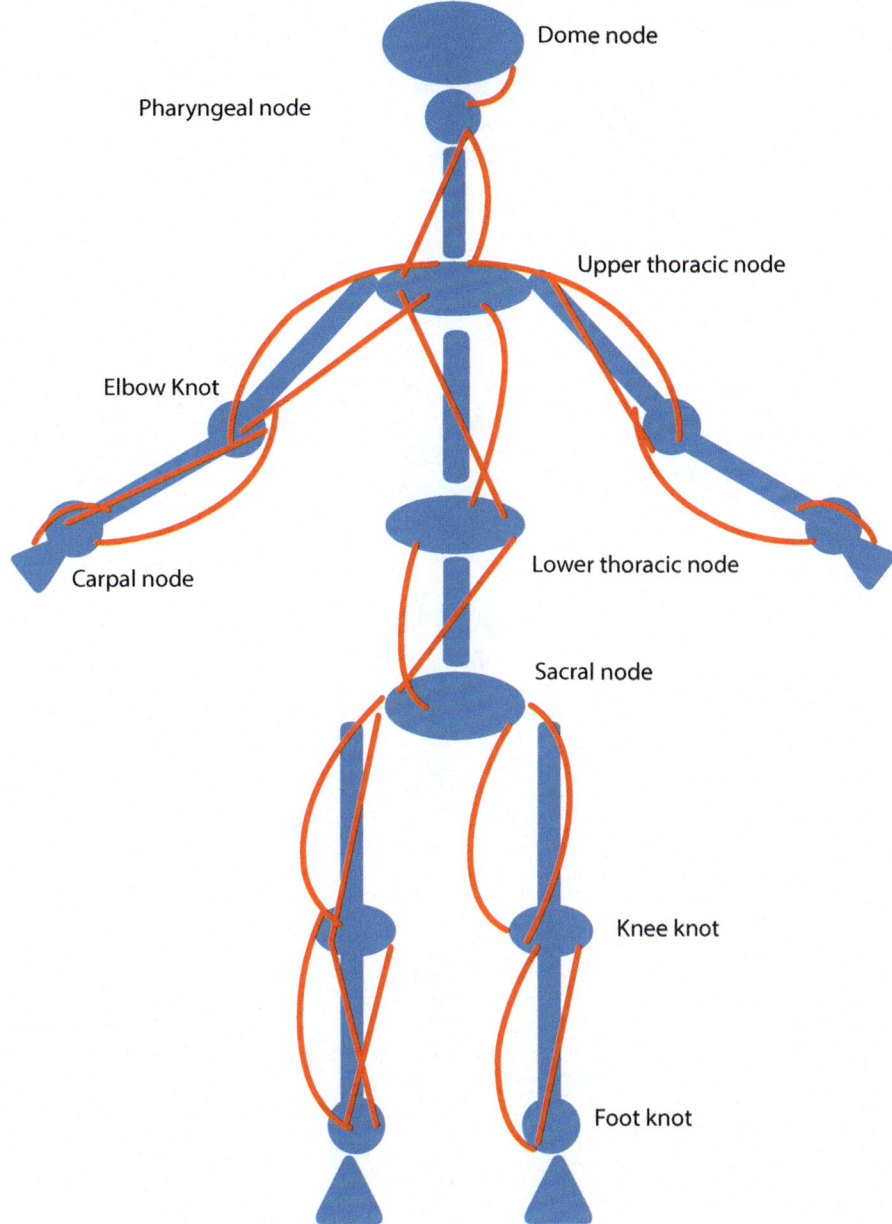

Fig. 3.7 Course of the most important fascial chains in the frontal plane

Hypertensions then also lead to periosteal reactions, such as in tennis elbow or directly to tension-related mispositioning of bones. This would correspond to the legendary "jumped out" vertebra. On the skull, said tension stress leads to headaches. However, hypertension can also have other consequences. Tensions on

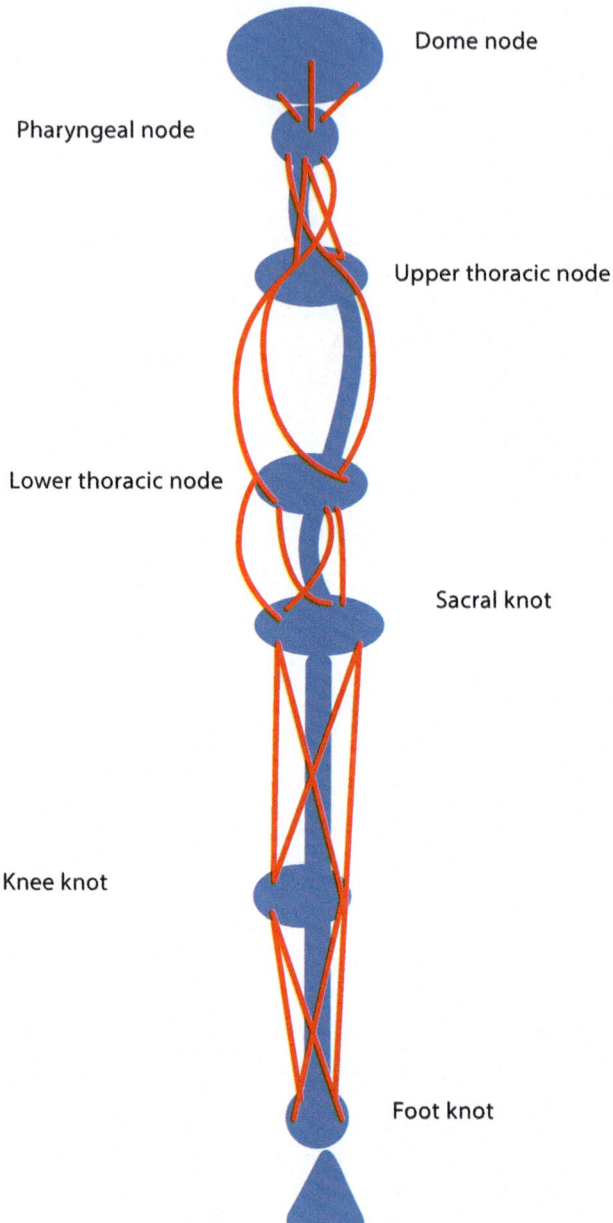

Fig. 3.8 Course of the most important fascial chains in the sagittal plane

the petrous bone, usually triggered by tension on the mastoid, lead to direct disturbances of the inner ear with the result of vertigo and hypacusis. It is important to recognize that all connections of the body are dynamic and mobile. Even a skull suture is not rigid. Tension stress on the petrous bone has consequences and disturbs the function of the labyrinth and the cochlea. In a lecture of mine, an orthopedist was completely astonished at how I could consider the sacroiliac joint to be complexly mobile. For him, it was simply a rigid, static connection. However, there are no such things in nature. Everything is dynamic and permeable. Just consider that even a skyscraper must be capable of oscillating. How much more must dynamics be the principle of a moving organism.

The sources of disturbance in the myofascial organ have somatic components, such as swelling, lymphatic or venous congestion, for example in inflammations (dental foci, sinusitis, prostatitis). Or also altered organ structures, which inhibit the body's dynamics with reduced glideability. Examples of this would be restrictive ventilation disorders, steatosis hepatis, hypersplenism, kidney cysts, pericardial effusions, hypertrophic heart diseases, myomas, etc. Traumatic adhesions of myofascial compartments, such as surgical scars, are also among the somatic triggers of myogeloses (= blockages).

However, even more common are the psycho-neurological causes that cause a generalized increase in tone of the myofascial organ (see Fig. 3.3).

Thus, anxiety disorders, depressions and distress are always associated with blockages, mostly in the area of psychomotor skills, i.e., in the pharyngeal or calotte node. These then often lead to complaints at other nodes via activation of fascial chains.

The following diagrams show the analysis of 500 male and 500 female treatment cases of different patients from the first three quarters (January to September) 2018 in my consultation, broken down by the cause of the myofascial syndrome. In addition, I show the distribution of symptoms in both collectives.

The selected patients had to be between 20 and 60 years old and have at least one of the following diagnoses:

Myogelosis, blockage, tension headache, pain, migraine, lumbago, neck-shoulder-arm syndrome, insertion tendopathy.

The numbers behind the symptom-causing organs are in percent, with the sum of the numbers being greater than 100% because some patients had several causes for the painful myofascial syndromes (Figs. 3.9 and 3.10).

Striking is the large number of psychosomatic causes as triggers for myofascial syndromes in both groups, with women leading slightly. Dental diseases are also common, often representing pressure-induced, aseptic jaw osteitis, which are ultimately caused by increased bite tone—mostly at night—and then again belong to psychogenic disorders.

The experienced therapist must therefore always examine the structures in the pharyngeal node, for this one must also palpate the Mm. pterygoidei intraorally. Often, these patients also show abrasions of the teeth and report sleep disorders. It is typical here that affected patients wake up between 1 and 2 o'clock at night and then only sleep restlessly and fragmented. In addition, when considering the genesis of sleep disorders and bruxism, one must always think of atopies. The reduced nocturnal endogenous corticoid levels cause an increase in atopic mediators such as histamine and prostaglandins, which have a sleep-disturbing effect.

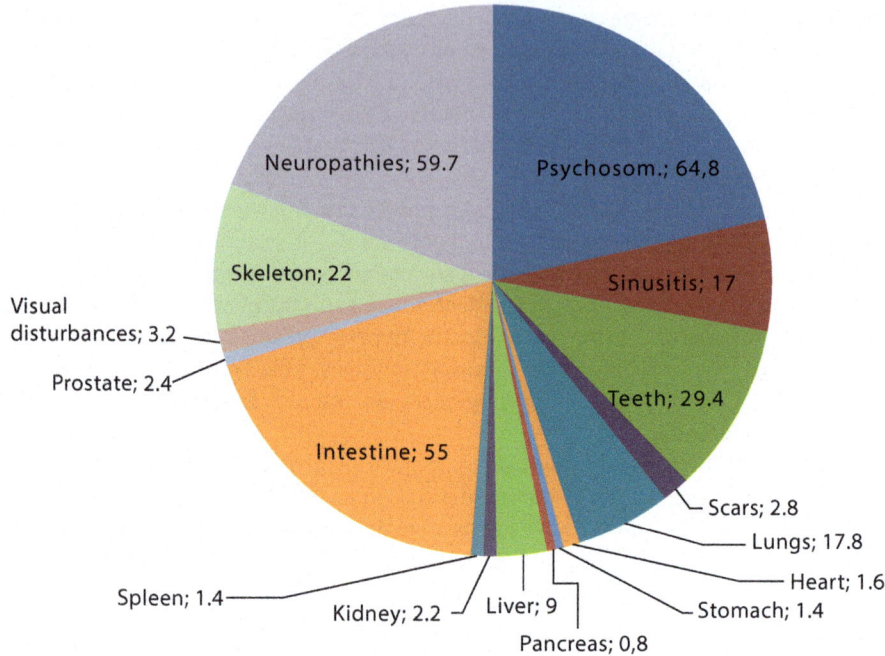

Fig. 3.9 Men (20–60 years, n = 500), information in % of cases

Especially in children, this is very common and often the only symptom of an allergy. These children are usually behaviorally conspicuous, unfocused and unbalanced in school. These symptoms can be easily managed with anti-allergic therapy.

Frequent intestinal disorders are also often of atopic nature or are due to intolerances to various sugars (lactose, etc.). The high sugar consumption in our society plays a significant role, as it leads to changes in the microbiome. Dysbiosis then often results directly in allergic disorders, food intolerances, and functional intestinal disorders, such as irritable bowel syndromes, chronic constipation, and meteorism. In particular, an overinflated colon transversum directly affects the lower thoracic node.

The frequency of allergic disorders also explains the frequency of sinusitis as a myogelosis-triggering disease.

In men, the frequency of lung and liver diseases should be mentioned, which probably has its cause in an unhealthier lifestyle. Lung function then usually shows restrictive ventilation disorders, often with significantly reduced ventilation capacity. The liver in these patients is usually significantly fatty, which can be quickly diagnosed using a sonogram.

Ultrasound is also the non-plus-ultra of diagnostics for other organ diseases. Pericarditis, pericardial effusions, hypertrophied myocardium, upper abdominal

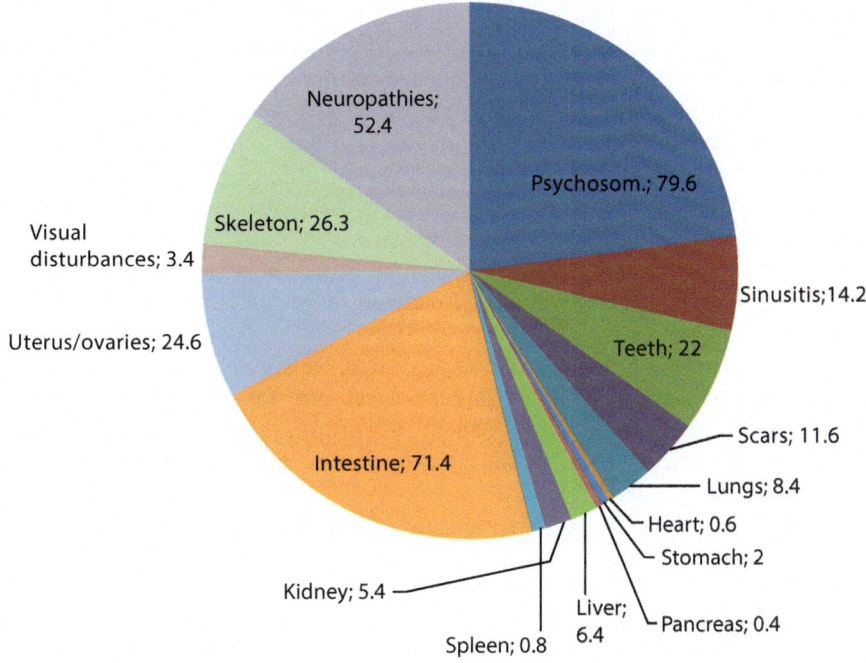

Fig. 3.10 Women (20–60 years, n = 500), information in % of cases

and renal pathologies, as well as prostate, uterus, and ovarian changes can be easily detected with it.

Women often develop blockage symptoms due to scars and adhesions in the small pelvis, usually after cesarean births or other gynecological surgeries.

Of course, skeletal triggers also account for an important proportion of the causes of myofascial syndromes, with about 22 and 26.3%. However, overall, I find their significance surprisingly low. Many patients with post-traumatic leg length differences, spinal fusions, scoliosis, arthrosis, etc., have very few fascial problems. Of course, arthrosis also leads to myogelosis. However, they are easy to recognize and usually less problematic to treat with physiotherapy and modern prosthetics than expected.

I very often see patients with functional leg length differences or gonarthrosis who are orthopedically treated with length-compensating or axis-adjusting insoles. I usually experience these insoles as fatal because they oppose dynamic-functional compensation and cause a lot of damage. Insoles must always be functional as long as this is possible. By "functional," I mean that they must activate muscular mechanisms that lead to motor support or, in the case of the foot, to the erection of the disturbed arches. This applies especially to foot arch disorders in children, who should always be treated with physiotherapy. Only older patients may benefit from pure support.

In general, I believe that supportive measures, such as bandages, orthoses, or even corsets, are completely counterproductive in the treatment of myofascial symptoms. This also applies to consequences at peripheral nodes, such as tendovaginitis in the forearm or insertion tendopathies.

For some time now, I have had my practice in a large home for people with disabilities. Therefore, I treat many patients with infantile cerebral palsy who have had the worst asymmetric spasticity since early childhood and have consequently developed severe skeletal deformities.

These patients were previously provided with rigid seat or lying shells to catch the deformities. This often leads to an increase in general spasticity with severe pain.

As far as possible within our insurance system, we are moving away from shell care towards dynamic bedding in fabrics, which are, for example, incorporated into wheelchairs. This care allows patients to perform rotating movements in the body axis, which leads to a significant reduction in muscle spasticity and much less pain for the patients.

Neuropathic problems are important and relatively frequent. In our area, neuroborreliosis is particularly common.

I also count the often overlooked angle anomalies among neurological problems. This refers to axis deviations of the eyes, which often do not manifest as strabismus. These patients usually "squint" only when they are tired, but also have double vision from time to time, leading to alternating—often alternating—shutdown of one eye. The patients therefore see in two dimensions only in phases.

They often report constantly bumping into things and having difficulty reading. Children often have serious school problems because reading is much more strenuous for them than for children whose axis coordination works without restrictions. These patients very often suffer from tension headaches up to migraines.

I have to digress briefly about migraines. Certainly, the myofascial organ is closely involved in their genesis. In any case, many patients can be helped well through relaxing measures. Manipulative techniques initially have no sustainability because the triggering of the migraine attack occurs centrally. The disturbances usually originate from the calotte and pharyngeal nodes and are often psychogenically triggered. Hypertension of the psychomotor muscles and direct hypertension in the myofascial organ probably play an important role, with the release of inflammatory mediators, such as calcitonin gene-related peptide (CGRP), also occurring. I always combine physiotherapeutic therapy immediately with tricyclic antidepressants, triptans, rarely beta-blockers, or calcium antagonists, never antiepileptics, but increasingly with cannabinoids. All these substances act on the central nervous trigger of migraines, which I consider a myogelotic disorder. Cannabinoids, in particular, show astonishing success. By the way, also in fibromyalgia syndrome. My good friend Nemath Fazli, a neurologist, recently expressed the idea that fibromyalgia is a generalized form of migraine. His suspicion that CGRP antibodies, which help with migraines, also work in fibromyalgia, seems to be proving true.

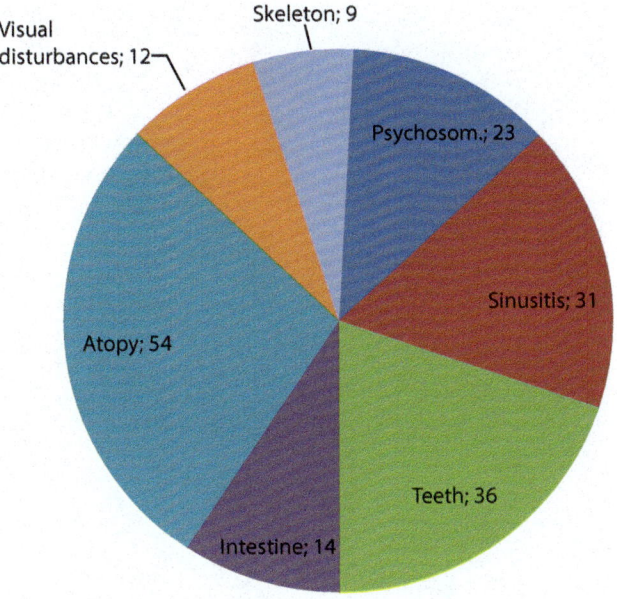

Fig. 3.11   Children (5-14 years, n = 100), information in % of cases

The two diseases are thus very similar and, in my opinion, are a disorder of the myofascial organ with a central—often post-traumatic—cause.

In daily practice, myofascial, holistic therapy approaches can certainly help 80% of migraine patients significantly.

Since I treat many children, here is an analysis from my practice. It refers to 100 treated children aged 5 to 14 years from four quarters in 2017. Here, too, there were multiple diagnoses (Fig. 3.11). Blockages are also common in children. The often-cited "growing pain" is, of course, actually a myofascial event. It often occurs in the context of growth spurts because functional, motor misalignments usually occur here—probably because our brain has to learn to control a now larger body. Of course, psychogenic disorders in children are also becoming more frequent. Atopies play an enormous role, as described for adults. Specific to children, however, are the myogeloses triggered by braces, which very often manifest themselves in tension headaches or symptoms at other nodes. I also see parasitic intestinal diseases almost weekly in my practice. They are difficult to diagnose but are characterized by the clinic. Regular abdominal problems with lumbago, knee, or foot pain are typical. It is then often better to treat "blindly" with an anthelmintic than to attempt diagnostics. Finally, I would like to address the frequent and easily overlooked Pelvic-Congestion- Syndrome, which affects about 15% of women over 40 and usually manifests itself through persistent myogeloses with lumbago, groin, and tension headaches—typically after prolonged sitting. It is understood to be a varicose condition of the ovarian and uterine veins, leading to congestion in the small pelvis. Fig. 3.12 shows a typical finding.

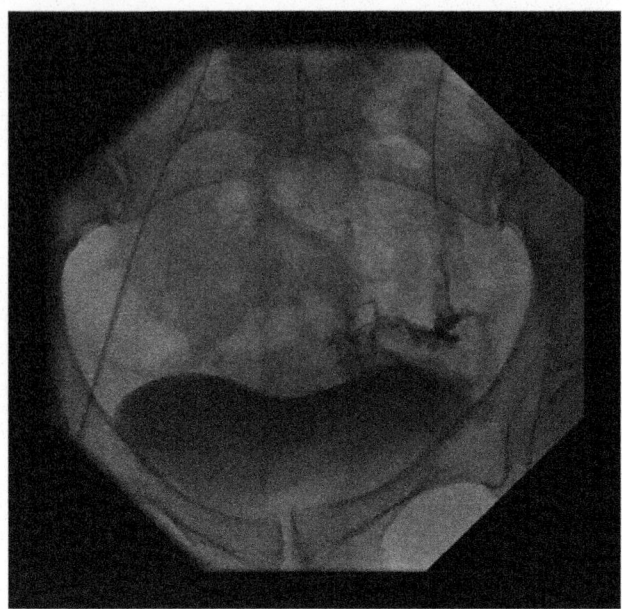

Fig. 3.12 Varicose veins on the right ovary of a 40-year-old patient with long-standing groin pain

Clinical Presentation of Myofascial Syndromes

4

Contents

The illustrations in this chapter show the most common symptoms of blockages or myogeloses at the individual nodes. All these disorders provide no other physical findings, except for the palpable myogeloses. These do not always cause active pain, their consequences are manifold, but initially always only functional. A blockage-related otalgia, for example, exists without any other abnormalities in the middle ear—except perhaps a non-irritating effusion due to poor ventilation, visual disturbances exist without somatic findings in the eye. Arthralgias show no abnormalities in laboratory or imaging procedures. Myogelotic complaints initially always lack somatic findings. Only when they persist for a longer period, damage occurs, such as tendinoses with calcifications, etc.

Following the list of node-specific complaints, there is always the distribution of the mentioned symptoms of my patients in a pie chart. For this purpose, I have examined the data of 100 patients aged 20 to 60 years, who showed disorders in the respective node, without differentiating by gender. Due to multiple symptoms, the sum of the percentages is again over 100%.

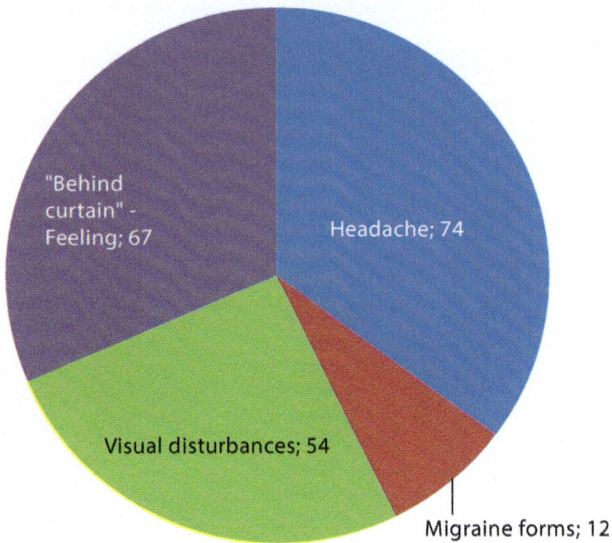

Fig. 4.1 Percentage distribution of symptoms KK

4.1   Calotte Node

- Headaches, migraine pain with light/sound sensitivity,
- Visual disturbances, which mostly produce changing spots or shadows in the visual field, mouches volantes, focusing problems
- The feeling of experiencing the world as if behind a curtain, not being able to think properly (Fig. 4.1)

4.2   Pharyngeal Node

- Ear pain, eustachian tube ventilation disorders
- Tinnitus
- Vertigo
- Sudden hearing loss
- Jaw pain, jaw lock
- Neck pain, limited mobility
- Feeling of a lump, swallowing disorders
- Hoarseness, laryngeal irritation cough
- Phonation disorders (Fig. 4.2)

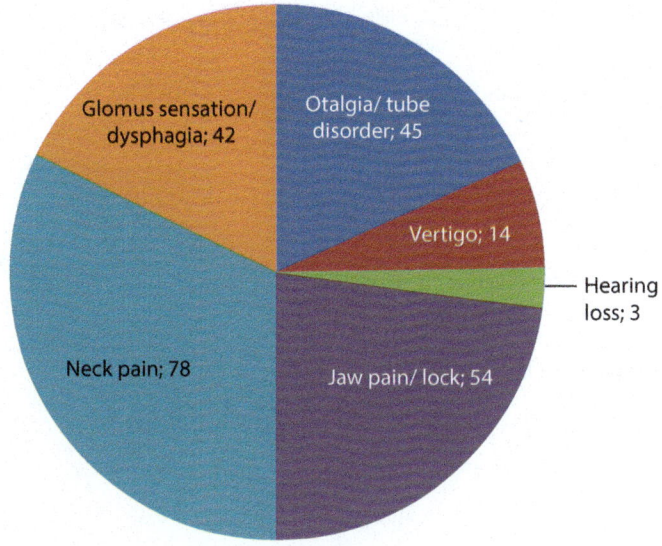

Fig. 4.2 Percentage distribution of symptoms PK

4.3   Upper Thoracic Node With Chain Into the Arm

- Shoulder pain of any kind and severity
- Restrictions in movement
- Paresthesia in the arm
- Arthralgia, insertion tendopathies, tennis elbow
- Restrictions in movement
- Tendovaginitis
- Swelling
- Intercostal neuralgia
- Breathing difficulties
- Angina-like complaints, which usually occur at rest
- Feeling of pressure (Fig. 4.3)

4.4   Lower Thoracic Node

- Breathing difficulties
- Pain in the lower thoracic area and upper lumbar spine, intercostal neuralgia
- Pressure sensations in the upper abdomen, often with agonizing nausea
- Gastralgia
- Feeling of fullness (Fig. 4.4)

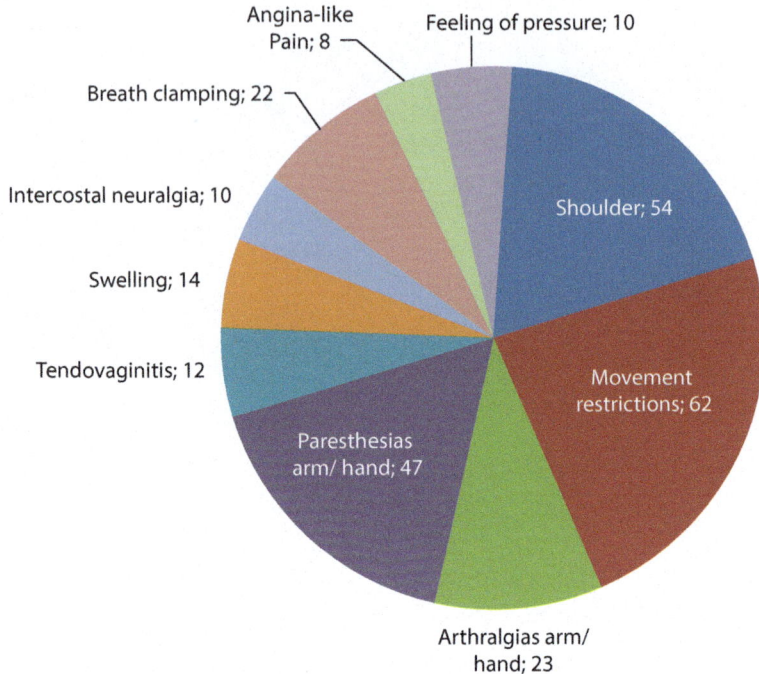

Fig. 4.3 Percentage distribution of OTK symptoms

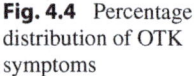 **Fig. 4.4** Percentage distribution of OTK symptoms

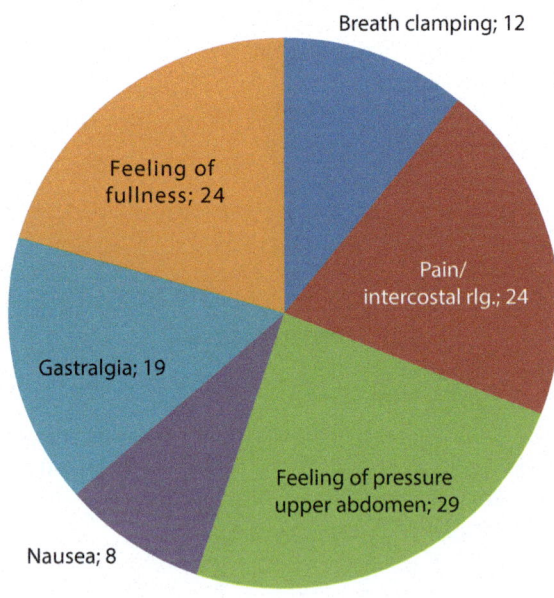

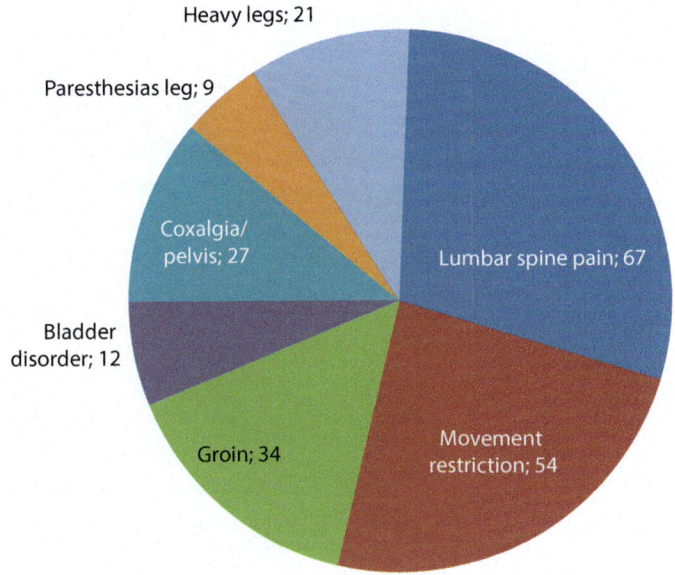

Fig. 4.5 Percentage distribution of symptoms in sacral node

4.5   Sacral Node

- Lower back pain, limited mobility
- Groin pain, groin swelling
- Scrotal pain
- Urinary urgency
- Bladder emptying disorders, often seen as overflow bladder in children
- Coxalgia, limited mobility and pain in pelvic muscles
- Paresthesia in the leg
- "Heavy legs", leg swelling
- Very often with myogelotic involvement of the M.tens. fasciae latae (Fig. 4.5)

For the peripheral nodes of the leg, I have omitted a breakdown of the symptom distribution because it is not particularly informative.

4.6   Knee Node

- Gonalgia, limited mobility
- Irritative effusions
- Promotion of muscle ruptures in the calf and thigh

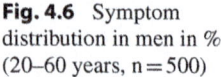

Fig. 4.6 Symptom distribution in men in % (20–60 years, n = 500)

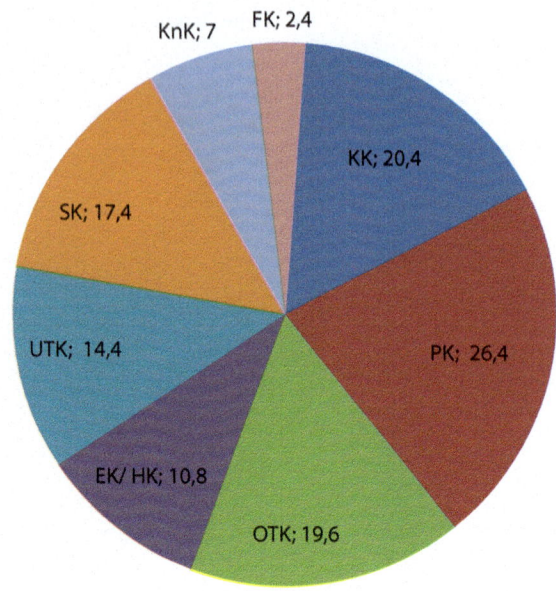

4.7   Foot Nodes

- Foot pain
- Achillodynia
- Foot swelling

The following diagrams show the distribution of symptoms on the nodes in the groups shown above. Due to multiple symptoms, the sum of the percentages is greater than 100 (Figs. 4.6 and 4.7).

As the two pie charts show, there are few significant differences between men and women. Men suffer slightly more often from disorders of the upper thoracic node, mostly shoulder pain and arm symptoms. While women more often suffer from symptoms of the calotte node, mostly headaches. Women also seem to be more susceptible to disorders in the sacral node, which is probably due to the much more complex anatomy of the small pelvis (Fig. 4.8).

In children, symptoms in the lower extremities occur much more frequently than in adults, but they show fewer symptoms in the KK or PK.

Fig. 4.7 Symptom distribution in women in % (20–60 years, n = 500)

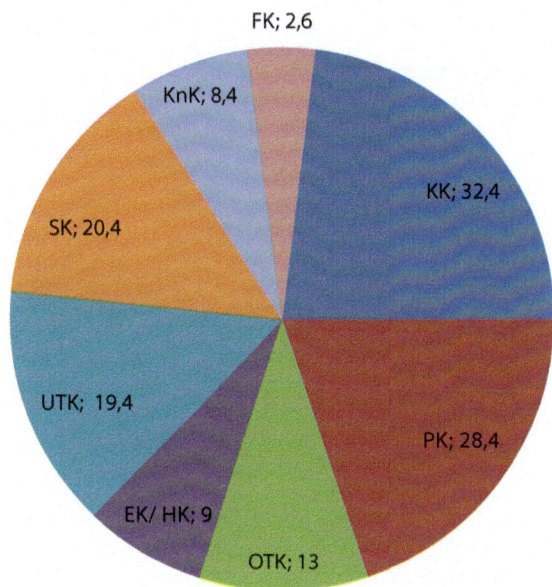

Fig. 4.8 Symptom distribution in children in % (5–14 years, n = 100)

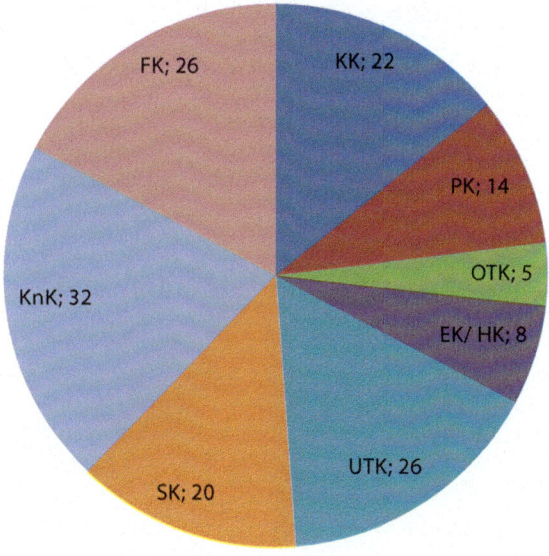

General Medical Diagnostic and Treatment Approaches

5

Contents

It would actually be urgently necessary to convey much more knowledge about the myofascial organ in medical studies. With a wink, I would say that one could abolish the subject of orthopedics and replace it with "myofasciology." Students should also learn much more about manual therapy techniques. It would be desirable to have joint training sections with physiotherapy schools. I started with chiropractic at the age of 18, during my civilian service, by seeking teachers myself. The techniques I learned back then often helped me more in everyday clinical practice than many of the other areas I learned during my studies.

Since most practicing colleagues lack manual therapy experience, I will not describe this in this chapter. This will be done further down.

Of course, the diagnosis begins with the anamnesis, which contributes 80% to the correct diagnosis.

Fluctuating pain, rest pain at varying times of the day, disturbances during activities, or other sensations, such as postprandial shortness of breath, etc., always provide an indication of a myogelotic event.

The suspicion is confirmed by the physical examination.

I pick up my patients in the waiting room and walk with them about 8 meters into a treatment room. Often there are already touches (hand on the shoulder or back). The following can be assessed:

- How does the patient appear: very burdened and stressed or smiling?
- How does he get up from the chair: easily, dynamically, or disharmoniously?
- What is the posture: shoulder tilt, hypodynamic spinal sections?
- How does the patient walk: upright-dynamic, uneven, disharmonious, wooden, or tensionless?
- How does the patient appear under a touch: soft, flexible, pleasant, or tense, adynamic, disharmonious?

After the anamnesis, which will be familiar to the reader, the physical examination follows.

I examine the calotte, pharyngeal, and upper thoracic nodes in the sitting patient, starting cranially.

I feel my way from the temporal region over the jaw, neck, throat to the shoulder and axillary region and take the Kibler's fold in the thoracic area, which works well even with clothed patients.

I examine the upper thoracic node by palpating from ventral to caudal along the lower thoracic aperture.

To examine the sacral node, I have the patient stand up, sit down on the examination stool behind the patient, and examine the abdominal and groin tension, the pelvic position, and the tension of the gluteal muscles.

If I find myogeloses or blockages in the upper nodes up to this point, I deblock them chiropractically and then continue to examine the lying patient.

First, I place the patients on their stomachs, deblock the lower thoracic area if necessary, and then examine the sacral node from caudal again.

Then the patient turns, and I check tensions in the thigh adductors, test abduction and adduction, as well as rotation in the hip joint.

After that, I place my thumbs on both inner ankles and observe leg length asymmetries while the patient sits up, which often only occur temporarily during movement.

Finally, I deblock the sacral node chiropractically if necessary.

The whole procedure takes about 5 minutes and provides the most important clues as to where to look more closely for pathologies. In addition, findings about skeletal anomalies, hyperkyphoses/lordoses, scolioses are obtained, which, however, usually cause fewer myofascial problems than suspected. Probably because postural anomalies are well compensated, especially if they develop slowly.

In the following organizational charts, it is shown how I then proceed. The method moves from the more common differential diagnoses to the rarer ones. Each organizational chart refers to a node. Skeletal disorders are not considered because their diagnosis is relatively simple and a general medical focus is applied here.

5.1 Calotte Node

In the calotte node, sinusitis is the most common cause of blockages. Anamnestic findings often include nocturnal nasal obstruction with mouth breathing. Children often snore. By the way, sleep apnea syndromes also often lead to myogeloses but can be easily diagnosed via polysomnography.

If sinusitis is found, I always treat it first. Methason-containing nasal sprays are very helpful in this case. If necessary, I also resort to oral cortisone shock therapy (I almost never need antibiotics here). If success is not achieved, a CT scan of the paranasal sinuses is needed to possibly subject polyps, cysts, etc. to surgery.

Angular deviations can also be easily recognized. To do this, I put Yoked Prism Glasses (= spatial displacement glasses, the term probably originates from the first impression of the person who used such glasses to test the visual and postural flexibility: they felt like being under a "yoke") on the patient, which distort the surroundings so that the patient can no longer access optical, central experience values. Patients with one eye "switched off" can then no longer walk in a straight line. They become extremely unstable and stagger like drunkards.

For more precise diagnostics and therapy, I send these patients to the optometrist and sometimes to the ophthalmologist. It is not enough for the affected patients to simply alternately blind one eye each, so that binocularity is maintained, but they must practice with their eyes. This is especially true after being fitted with axis-regulating prism glasses, then there is no visual deterioration, as is often proclaimed (Fig. 5.1).

To test inner ear functions simply with the means of general medicine, the Weber and Rinne test is still a brilliant instrument. It should be familiar to everyone.

For the rarer central diseases, which sometimes initially mimic symptoms of a myofascial syndrome, it is recommended to search for Lyme disease in the laboratory. MS, tumors, etc. require an MRI, sometimes also a lumbar puncture.

The treatment depends on the diagnosis.

5.2 Pharyngeal Node

In my experience, dental foci most frequently disturb the PK, whereby I also consider a pressure-induced jaw osteitis with increased bite tone as a dental focus. With a bite force of approximately 800 N/cm^2, pressure-loaded teeth are literally lowered by aseptic jaw bone resorption.

In such cases, close cooperation with resourceful dentists is always required, who can often defuse asymmetries with minimal bite correction or achieve a lot with bite splints. It is very important that patients go to the bite adjustment in a deblocked state, because activated fascial chains shift the bite when myogeloses are present. I schedule patients directly before the dentist appointment or coordinate the visit with physiotherapists who deblock the patients beforehand.

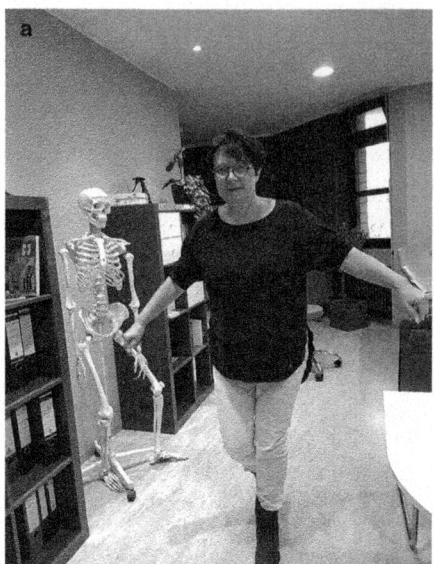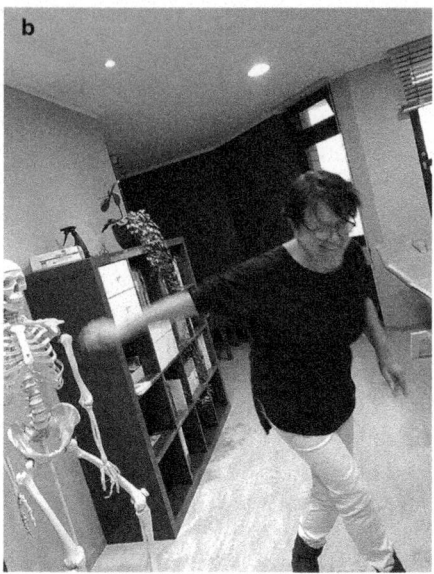

Fig. 5.1 Patient becomes completely unstable and staggers to the left when attempting to walk in a straight line with Yoked Prism Glasses

Treatment of depressive triggers is also essential. In addition to psychological methods, a tricyclic, such as Amitriptyline 12.5 to 50 mg or Opipramol 10 to 25 mg, sometimes also Mirtazapine 15 mg, is often very helpful for improving sleep architecture. Due to the low side effects, I also sometimes try Agomelatine 25 mg, a melatonin receptor agonist. Patients benefit quickly from these measures and report an improvement in myogeloses after just a few days. So, one does not have to treat for three weeks, as one would if treating with antidepressants.

Unfortunately, I see relatively frequent female patients—rarely men—with massive headache problems or severe myofascial pain syndromes, who mostly come with the diagnosis of migraine or fibromyalgia and have always undergone countless therapies. Many of these patients have experienced sexual abuse in childhood and often develop their symptoms only at the age of 30. Since the prescription of cannabinoids is finally possible, there is finally the opportunity to help these patients. I always use THC-containing oils; in my opinion, CBD is less crucial here.

Unilateral cerumen, e.g., in divers, ear canal eczema, or anatomical variations, can also trigger massive myogeloses with, for example, tension headaches.

Chronic laryngeal irritation in the sinubronchial syndrome, reflux, or atopy also affects the myofascial organ, which is not surprising given the complexity of the anatomical laryngeal suspension and the corresponding neurological control.

5.3   Upper Thoracic Node

As already described, it is mostly the organ-compliance-altering diseases that lead to blockages. Therefore, myogeloses are less common in asthma than in restrictive lung diseases. Heart diseases are rather rare in patients under 60.

5.4   Lower Thoracic Node

Due to the significant influence of the intestine with its glands (liver/pancreas) in the UTK, intestinal disorders must be in focus.

A huge problem here is the sugar consumption in our society, which, together with the frequent and often unnecessary antibiotic therapies, leads to a depletion of the intestinal flora. Much has been and is being written about this, and the findings are fascinating. I consider the microbiome of the intestine as a separate organ, which, just like the kidney, liver, etc., belongs to our body with its function.

Intestinal rehabilitations are often very important, but also difficult. Fasting cures or probiotics often do not help sustainably, which is probably also due to a secretory milieu disturbance of the mucosa.

I developed a simple food pyramid for my type II diabetics 21 years ago, which I now recommend to all patients because it has proven to be excellent.

The key to success probably lies in the reduction of carbohydrates, the high fiber and plant content, and—quite essential—the introduction of a "treat day". Only on the said treat day are there sweets, such as jam, honey, juices, and everything that tastes sweet. Sugar thus becomes more of a pleasure product. However, I always advise my patients with a wink to cultivate as many different vices in moderation as possible. For some people, compensating for a "sugar flush" with hot peppers is also very helpful. Capsaicin activates our endorphin system[1] and relaxes, like chocolate (Fig. 5.2).

Very often, women around the age of 40 suddenly develop food intolerances, histamine intolerances, and allergic disorders with a luteal insufficiency. This is probably mainly due to the anti-allergic, cortisone-like effect of progesterone. In addition, estrogen and progesterone seem to promote the gene expression of histaminases. If there is a deficiency, women often cannot tolerate histamine-containing foods, such as aged cheese, smoked fish, or red wine anymore. The affected patients then report that they always felt particularly well during pregnancies. In this case, it is always worth trying a treatment with progesterone, e.g., 100 mg in the evening. Herbal remedies, such as Mexican wild yam extracts or Agnus Castus, can also be helpful. If the symptoms cannot be treated in this way, an appropriate pill must be used, with treatment often only lasting 6 months to a year, as the disorders then disappear on their own.

---

[1] This study was supported by Medical Research Institute Grant (2007–01), Pusan National University.

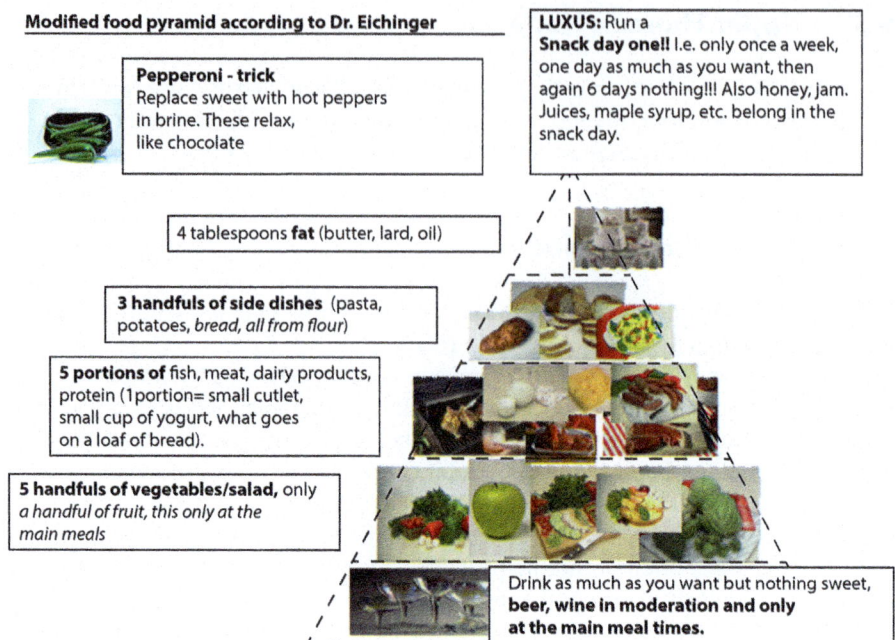

Modified food pyramid according to Dr. Eichinger

Pepperoni - trick
Replace sweet with hot peppers in brine. These relax, like chocolate

LUXUS: Run a **Snack day one!!** I.e. only once a week, one day as much as you want, then again 6 days nothing!!! Also honey, jam. Juices, maple syrup, etc. belong in the snack day.

4 tablespoons **fat** (butter, lard, oil)

3 handfuls of side dishes (pasta, potatoes, *bread, all from flour*)

5 portions of fish, meat, dairy products, protein (1portion= small cutlet, small cup of yogurt, what goes on a loaf of bread).

5 handfuls of vegetables/salad, only *a handful of fruit, this only at the main meals*

Drink as much as you want but nothing sweet, **beer, wine in moderation and only at the main meal times.**

You can calmly eat the entire contents of the Pytamide in one day without gaining weight. **It is very important to spread the food over 3 meals!!!** Between meals (4-5 hours break) you must not **eat anything or drink anything sweet.** You would otherwise raise your Insulin level, which leads to the total blockade of fat loss.
Allergy sufferers must pay attention to a healthy intestinal flora. Here, any sugar (even fructose) disturbs.

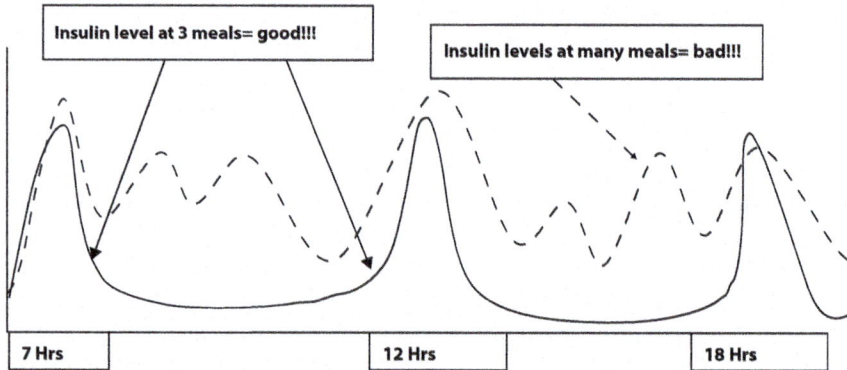

Insulin level at 3 meals= good!!!

Insulin levels at many meals= bad!!!

| 7 Hrs | 12 Hrs | 18 Hrs |

Fig. 5.2 Dietary recommendation, which is explained and handed out to my patients

5.5   Sacral Node

In the sacral node, postoperative scar disorders play a particularly important role. In the presence of external scars, an injection with a local anesthetic should always be attempted, which, similar to trigger point therapy, probably temporarily blocks pathological afferents of the scar connective tissue and thus causes a normalization of the myofascial tone. With regular therapy and mobilizing manipulation on the scar, our CNS seems to "subtract" it from the myofascial control.

I usually use Bubivacain because it lasts longer than Lidocain or Xylocain.

In case of suspected adhesions in the small pelvis, laparoscopy is sometimes unavoidable. However, the successes achieved through adhesiolysis are often astonishing.

5.6   Peripheral Nodes (EK, HK, KnK, FK)

The diagnostic clarification of peripheral nodes is relatively simple. Of course, relevant arthroses must be excluded as local disturbances, especially at the knee and thumb saddle joint.

Sometimes it is helpful to block afferents from joints with dexamethasone/xylocaine intra-articularly. If this leads to a rapid, significant improvement of myogeloses, it indicates an arthrotic process. If there is no improvement in existing arthroses, the wear and tear is not the problem of the blockade symptoms.

And foot arch disorders must also be treated physiotherapeutically or with functional insoles. Otherwise, as already mentioned, blockages of the periphery are usually the result of disturbances at central nodes.

Therapy of the Myofascial Organ

6

In addition to determining the causes and therapy of the same, manual therapeutic interventions are at the forefront of treating myofascial syndromes and complaints.

Many patients recover after a chiropractic or physiotherapeutic treatment. In this group, the complaints are usually triggered by monotonous, motor-neuronal stress. Typical examples are painting work, which always requires the same movement - often for hours - or forced postures, such as when "shifting in bed."

If patients initially experience a significant improvement after a deblocking therapy but then a resurgence of symptoms, triggering causes, as described in Chap. 4, must be found. If these are not treated, all manual therapeutic measures will not be sustainable.

By the way, all therapy effects must always be clear. It is helpful to have the patient rate the degree of discomfort on a visual analog scale from 0 to 10. An improvement of only one to two points is more likely due to a placebo effect.

For the general practitioner, among the manual therapy forms, chiropractic is the best method because it can be performed quickly and is very effective.

As with all manipulations, the activation of Ruffini-corpuscles and Golgi tendon organs in muscle and connective tissue is probably at the forefront, causing relaxation of the myofascial organ via reflex arcs. The idea of mechanically bringing collagen fibers into "shape" seems far-fetched to me. One cannot mechanically massage a spastic muscle soft or reduce a dislocation against muscle tension as long as no neurogenic relaxation of the structures has occurred. Manual therapeutic methods certainly improve the mobility between the layers of the myofascial organ mechanically. However, the main effect on the fiber itself is also more neurological-reflexive. It remains to be discussed whether the semi-liquid "gel" in which collagen fibers are embedded can also switch between sol and gel phases in a controlled manner - or perhaps behaves in a controlled manner like a dilatant dispersion, which alternates between liquid and viscous (the principle is used in shock absorbers). This would explain the gelosis, which usually disappears immediately after manipulation.

The chiropractic manipulation initially generates a mostly rotating tension, which ends in a short stretching impulse. This seems to me to cause a neurological-reflexive relaxation of the myofascial structures. The often rotatory component of tension and impulse seems to excite crossing afferents, which apparently is more neurologically efficient.

The observation is also supported by the fact that rotating gymnastic exercises efficiently relax more than unilateral movements. As mentioned above, I also see this in my patients with severe spasticity. Allowing rotational movements in positioning often significantly reduces spasticity. Hypertensive myofascial patterns are probably better broken up by the activation of crossing reflex arc afferents and efferents as well as effects on both hemispheres than if the activation only works unilaterally. Although the efficiency of chiropractic therapy is clear, it remains a symptomatic therapy that is usually limited to the treatment of nodal areas because this is where most blockages are located. It is not correct to assume that chiropractic therapy would "wear out" ligaments and joints if used too frequently. Of course, chiropractic therapy does not cause overstretching of the aforementioned structures. However, if a patient has complaints again immediately after therapy, further constant chiropractic intervention is unsatisfactory, and the physiotherapist should definitely be involved in the treatment. The fear of mechanical dissection of the intima media of the carotids during manipulations on the neck with the consequence of strokes is low if the therapy is gentle. There seem to be patients who are prone to such dissections (Wallenberg syndrome), but I have never encountered this after chiropractic therapy. I even have a patient who regularly came and comes for chiropractic therapy, who had a TIA when a friend hugged her tightly around the neck. In my opinion, chiropractic therapy is harmless if you gently manipulate following the concept of manipulation on the myofascial organ. Those who think they are "adjusting vertebrae" should be more cautious.

Physiotherapeutic intervention often does not occur on the painful, stretched fascial chain, but on the compressed opposite side.

Manipulation on the compressed side probably triggers a tension afference via Ruffini corpuscles and Golgi tendon organs, leading to the detonicization of the painful fascial chain.

Similar effects are achieved with tape therapies. These also activate tension afferents and probably relax through reflex mechanisms.

All measures should always be carried out in a relaxed manner and without great or even brutal force. Chiropractic therapy does not "realign" "dislocated vertebrae." All methods detonicize the tissue so that pseudoluxated structures return to their position on their own.

Thus, often immediately after manipulation, the elevated shoulder or functional leg length difference is eliminated, and the dislocated vertebra is correctly positioned again.

Cupping therapy also works on reflex arcs and tension sensors. It may also have mobilizing effects on fascial layers. "Detoxification mechanisms," as postulated by traditional medical forms, especially in "bloody" cupping, are doubtful. I have also never experienced a patient who would have benefited more from this therapy than from other manual approaches.

The same applies to the detoxifying effect of oils. Certainly, they do not bind "toxins" through the skin, as is often claimed in esoteric models, but the myofascial organ is undoubtedly influenced by olfactory impressions. No sense is as closely linked to emotional memories as the sense of smell. Keep in mind that the olfactory nerve is a direct cranial nerve, meaning it is not switched. Its fibers go directly to the primary cerebral cortex, the amygdala, and the limbic system. Olfactory impressions thus have quick and direct access to centers of emotional evaluation of our environment. Emotional stimuli here directly trigger efferent vegetative reactions and can, of course, relax or tense the myofascial organ. Good scents relax, which is why oils used in therapy should smell pleasant.

Other "exotic" therapies, such as singing bowls, also have an effect, otherwise they would not last so long in therapy. Probably the vibrations of the vibrating metal bowls applied to the body act directly on the Pacini receptors, which trigger reflexive-relaxing reactions. Certainly, sounds also have a great influence on the myofascial organ, as do all pleasant sensory perceptions. Therefore, it is advisable to involve as many of the patient's senses as possible in the therapy.

In Fig. 6.1, the therapy forms are sorted by their approach points.

Future studies will show whether this view is correct.

The use of local anesthetics seems to work directly through anesthesia of nociceptors. I also usually treat the toned fascial chain by injecting trigger points or myogeloses directly. For this, I prefer Bubivacain over Xylocain because it has a long-lasting effect. I do not use Procain at all, as the substance often provokes allergic disturbances.

Very often, myogelotic symptoms are resolved after one or two chiropractic treatments and with the treatment of the triggering disorder. Recovery should ideally occur quickly, within a week, after the cause has been resolved. If this is not the case, the patient must also be treated with physiotherapy. I believe that persistent myogeloses, which continue to exist after the cause has been eliminated, are based on neurologically ingrained misregulations. The myogelosis is, so to speak, "learned." To correct this, chiropractic alone is not enough; these disorders must be normalized through mobilizing techniques and should then disappear within a maximum of 4 weeks. Unfortunately, there is still a "physiotherapeutic" image of physiotherapy among doctors. Classical gymnastics may promote muscle building in postoperative muscle atrophy, but it is unsuitable for the treatment of the myofascial organ. In the case of persistent myogeloses, the physiotherapist must apply manipulative techniques, with the patient being passive. In my practice, I prescribe "manual therapy" on 95% of the issued physiotherapy prescriptions, and

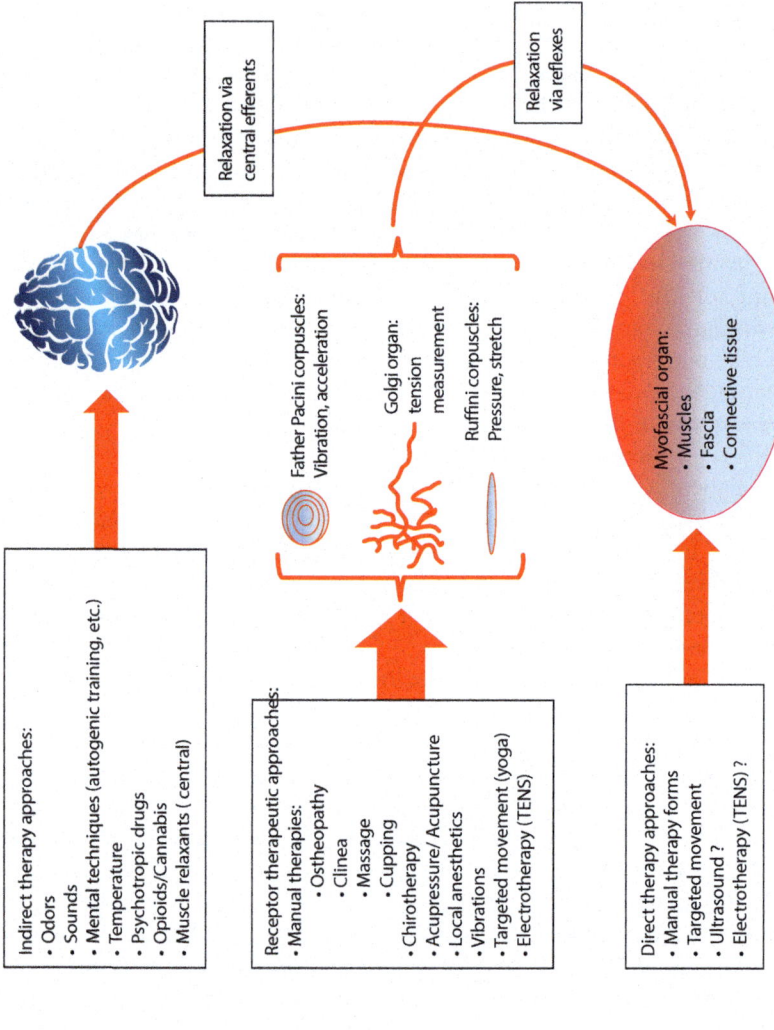

Fig. 6.1 Overview of therapy approaches to the myofascial organ

only a very small part of the patients need physiotherapy. Of course, a gymnastically trained, elastic musculoskeletal system is always beneficial in every respect, and gymnastics undoubtedly has a positive influence on the myofascial organ, but it brings little in the acute phase of a myofascial disorder.

Since it would be anachronistic in our multimedia world to describe techniques in prose and photos, we show all the procedures mentioned here on our website www.myofaszial.eu in videos.

Case Studies

7

Contents

7.1   Heterophoria

The following patient (*1971), farmer, positive Lyme serology, suffered from chronic back and knee pain for years. He often reported visual disturbances with floaters and the feeling of seeing through a veil. NMR LWS and knee did not yield a diagnosis.

In 2017, the patient was provided with prism glasses that compensate for the angular deviation in my practice by an experienced optometrist after a preliminary examination using Yoked Prism Glasses. Since then, the patient has been symptom-free.

Strangely enough, all three of his siblings had chronic symptoms with headaches and migraines. All three had heterophoria and were symptom-free after appropriate glasses were provided. It is absolutely necessary in optometric treatment to give patients exercises to shorten the central nervous adaptation phase to the new, three-dimensional visual impression, otherwise patients often have difficulty coping (Fig. 7.1).

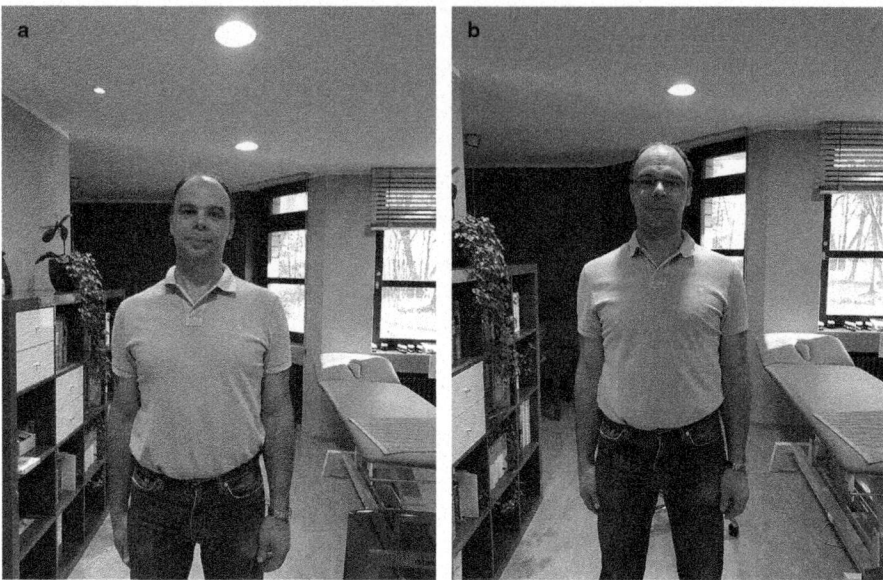

Fig. 7.1 The patient shows a significant shoulder misalignment to the right without glasses, with a lateral tilt of the head to the left. Both incorrect postures improve significantly simply by putting on the visual aid

7.2   "Growing Pains"

Very often, children with often severe pain come to my practice. The pain is often limited to the lower extremities. Of course, orthopedic conditions such as M. Perthes, M. Scheuermann, and hip cold must be considered, but usually a deblocking measure is sufficient to secure and treat the diagnosis of myogelosis (Figs. 7.2, 7.3 and 7.4).

7.3   Scar Disorder

The following patient (43 years old) has been suffering from chronic back pain since the extirpation of a liver hemangioma. Due to a simultaneous post-traumatic stress disorder after a rape at the age of 18, she developed a fibromyalgia syndrome with a chronic fatigue syndrome. At times, the patient took oxycodone 2×20 mg, which only resulted in insufficient pain reduction. Psychotherapy and antidepressants also provided no relief.

Ultimately, only consistent manual therapy with regular scar disorder treatments through mobilization and injection of local anesthetics proved helpful. The chronic fatigue syndrome improved significantly only after the use of a cannabinoid (dronabinol, 0–0–5 drops) (Fig. 7.5).

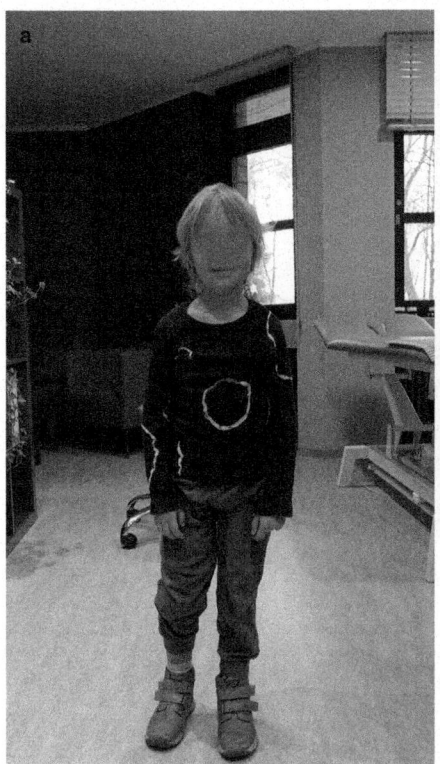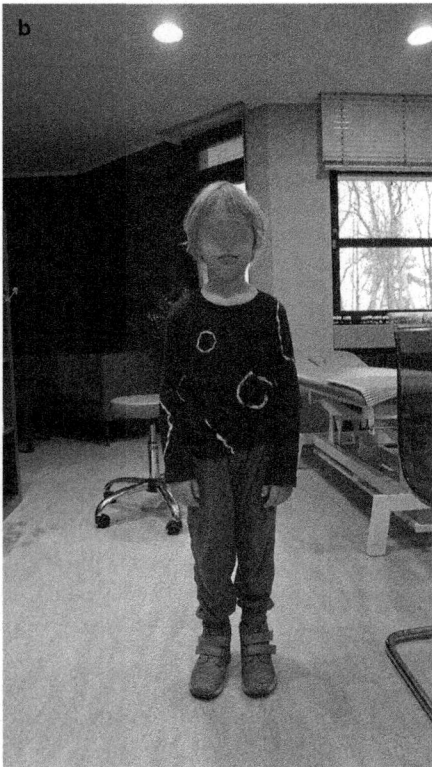

Fig. 7.2 This boy (6 years old) cannot bear weight on his right leg due to ankle pain that suddenly occurred after getting up. Blockages C2, C5, T1, L1, S1, and a temporomandibular joint blockage were then found. The cause was most likely psychosomatic, as the mother had started a rehabilitation measure for three weeks two days earlier. After a chiropractic deblocking, the weight can be immediately borne again, and the shoulder elevation is also better. The disturbance was due to hypertension of the fascial chain from PK during nocturnal bruxism via OTK (shoulder elevation) and finally SK with activation of the tensor fascia lat., which then led to the ankle pain. The patient was completely symptom-free after two hours

7.4 Dental Focus

An orthopantomogram (OPG) of a patient (72 years old) who had been suffering from pronounced Achilles tendon pain with swelling for 6 months is shown. The region had already been injected with corticosteroids from an orthopedic perspective, and he had also received insoles, which did not improve the situation. The corticosteroid injections only alleviated the symptoms for three to four days. Upon examination, a myogelosis in the PK over the right Mm. pterygoidei with a right lateral chain to the SK was revealed. Initiated manual therapy did not achieve lasting success, but at least improved the pain for five to six days. Since the symptoms

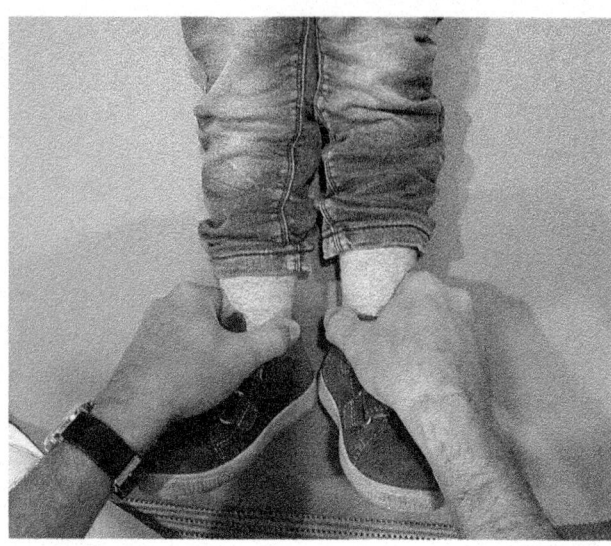

Fig. 7.3 This girl also complained of leg pain that suddenly occurred after getting up. She had grown significantly in recent weeks. Initially, there is a leg length difference of about 1 cm. To determine this, I simply place my thumbs on the two Maeolli med. and have the patient sit up. In the case of blockages, there is a functional leg length difference that must never be treated with "compensating" insoles, as these prevent equalizing control

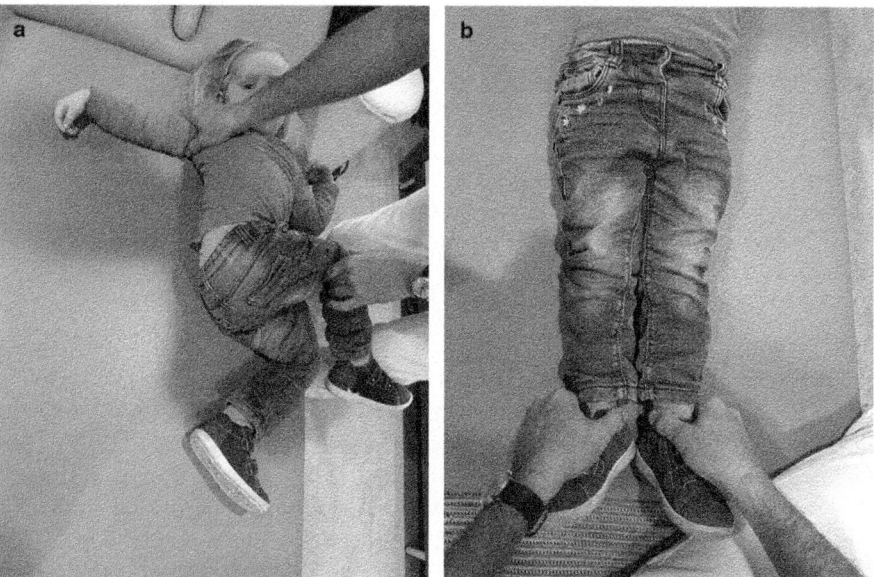

Fig. 7.4 Targeted deblocking of L4, S1. Immediate normalization of leg length difference afterwards

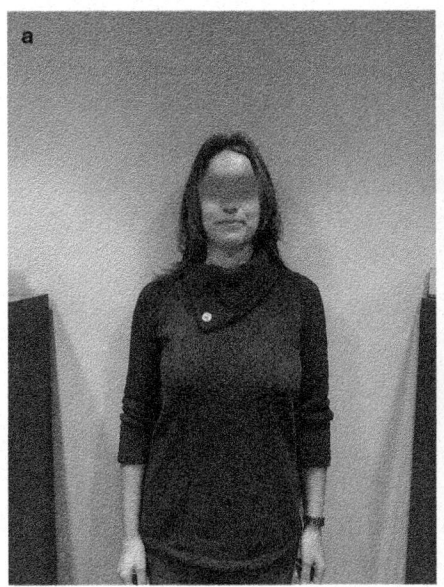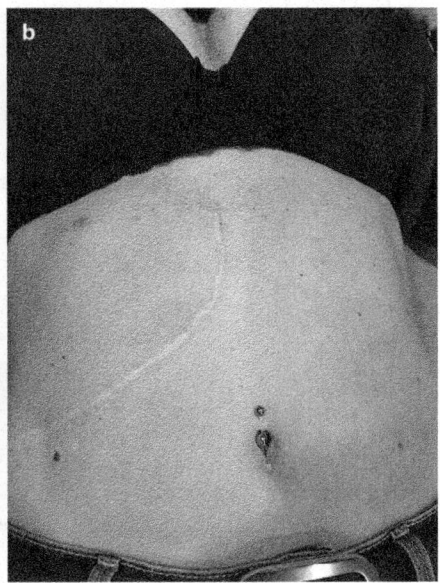

Fig. 7.5 Patient's incorrect posture with right shoulder depression, caused by the scar disorder in the lower thoracic spine with fascial chain downwards and upwards. On the right, the scar in the area of the lower thoracic spine

seemed to spread from the PK, I had an OPG made. Here, a focus was found on a root filling in the fourth quadrant.

In general, asymptomatic dental foci are often found on root fillings. This is due to the difficulty of treating a root canal in a sterile manner. I estimate the failure rate of root fillings, even with the best and most meticulous treatment, to be 20%. Since the affected teeth are denervated, there seems to be a lack of immunological defense. Typically, such foci cause tension headaches and often Achilles tendon pain and heel pain due to hypertension in the calf compartment and the plantar aponeurosis. After extraction of the affected tooth and the adjacent wisdom tooth, the patient was completely and sustainably pain-free after three sessions of physiotherapy. By the way, there is no side equality between dental focus and subsequent symptoms. Here, too, the focus was on the right, but the Achilles tendon pain was on the left (Figs. 7.6 and 7.7).

Dental foci do not necessarily have to be septic. Pressure loads during stress or bruxism also lead to jaw osteitis, because teeth are displaced away from the jaw under pressure. This displacement occurs through aseptic bone resorption, which also means jaw osteitis with its consequences on the myofascial organ. Patients with psychomotor problems and bruxism often show massive abrasions of the teeth (Fig. 7.8).

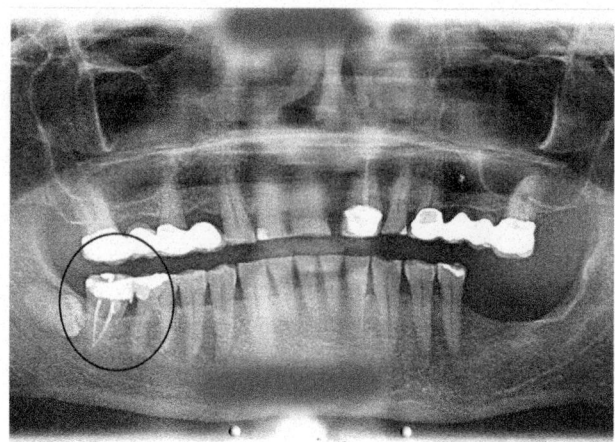

Fig. 7.6 Focus on tooth 47 with brightening around the root tip as a sign of a developing cyst. Next to it is also a wisdom tooth, which could be involved in the process

Fig. 7.7 Here the region is enlarged with the brightening around the tip at 47, as an expression of the jaw osteitis

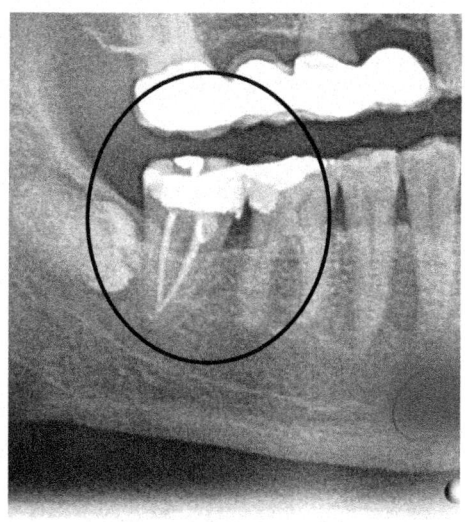

7.5   Ovarian Cyst

The following patient (55 years old) came limping with significant left-sided cox-algia, which had been present for two weeks, to the practice. A free hip joint was found, but there were isolated blockages in L1 to L5 and S1. This is always an indication of a disturbance in the sacroiliac joint (SIJ). The patient had a hyster-ectomy in 2015, which could result in adhesions that often lead to disturbances

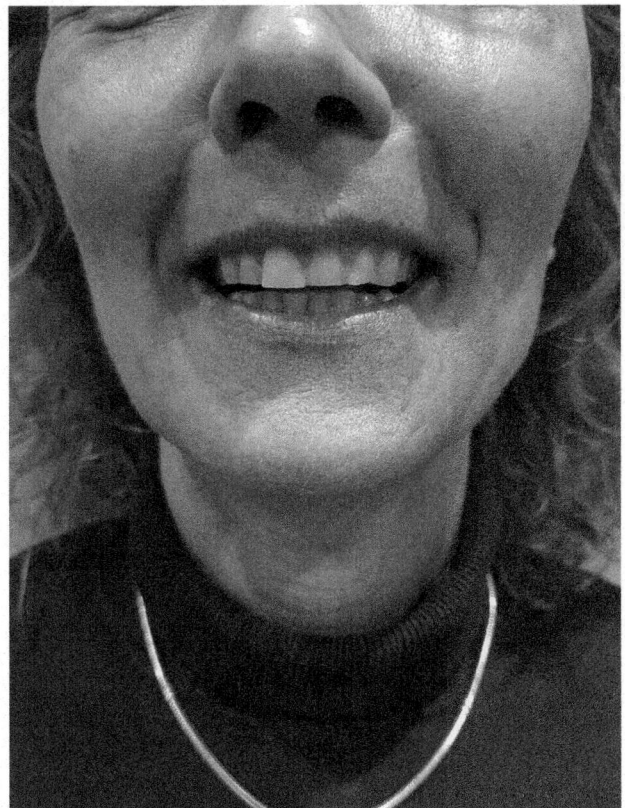

Fig. 7.8 Patient with chronic shoulder-arm syndrome and tendovaginitis on the right forearm. Massive abrasions are found. The canines are ground down to a line with the row of teeth. The patient benefited from Amitriptyline 12.5 mg at night and a bite splint, which distributed the nocturnal bite pressure somewhat better

in the SIJ and trigger myogeloses. In this patient, a 37 mm ovarian cyst with a clearly calcified ovary was found on ultrasound. After unblocking, the patient was symptom-free for a week, but then the myogelosis built up again. Only after laparoscopic oophorectomy was the patient persistently without symptoms (Figs. 7.9,7.10, and 7.11).

7.6 Jaw Misalignments

This girl (12 years old) came in with right ear pain. She had already been to a colleague the day before, who could not see the eardrum due to cerumen but prescribed an antibiotic as a precaution, which the mother had not given.

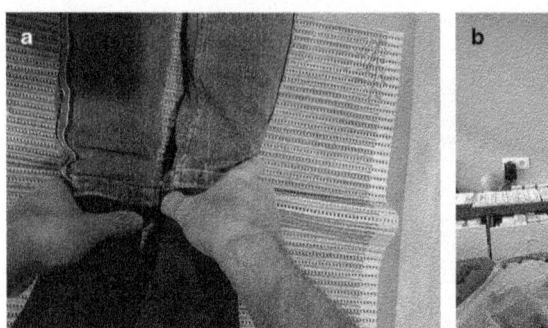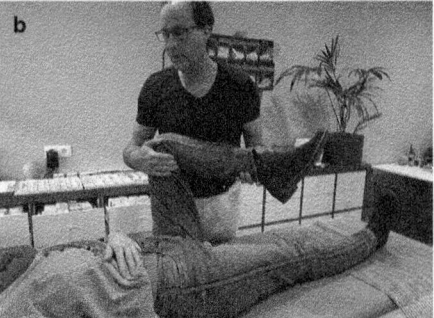

Fig. 7.9 Patient with approx. 2 cm leg length difference due to blockages in the SIJ. The hip appears free, although the complaints initially seem like the consequences of coxarthrosis

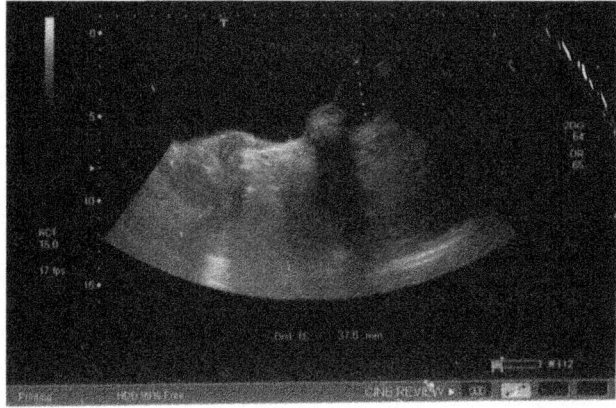

Fig. 7.10 Ultrasound shows a calcified ovary with a 37 mm cyst

After removal of the cerumen, an unirritated eardrum was revealed. The pronounced prognathism and elevated right shoulder were noticeable. Five days earlier, her braces had been adjusted (Fig. 7.12).

The examination then showed blockages in C2, C5, T1/2/3, and the right temporomandibular joint. These are common findings in orthodontic treatments. Often, children react with tension headaches or otalgia in the context of the adjustment in the PK.

After deblocking, especially of the chewing muscles, the ear pain disappeared immediately.

I also consider the importance of cerumen to be significant. A plug can indeed cause irritation in the PK and lead to vertigo, otalgia, and headaches (Figs. 7.13, 7.14, 7.15 and 7.16).

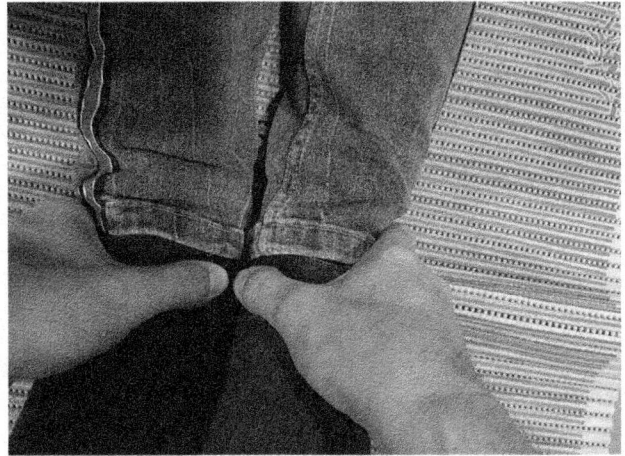

Fig. 7.11 After unblocking, the leg length difference is eliminated. Sustainability was only achieved in the patient after oophorectomy, with histology already showing cell atypia of the ovary

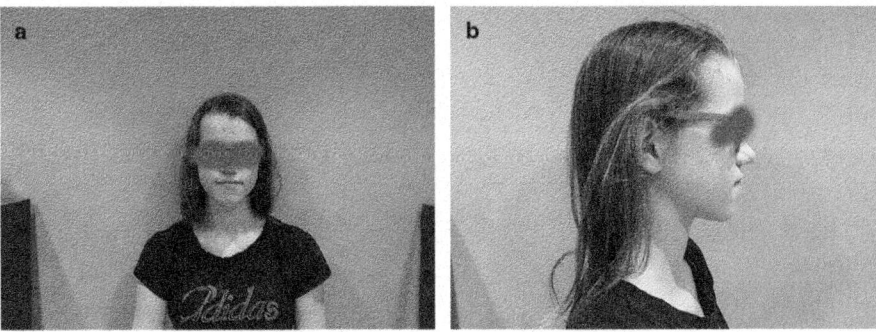

Fig. 7.12 Prognathism and elevated right shoulder with otalgia also on the right

62   7   Case Studies

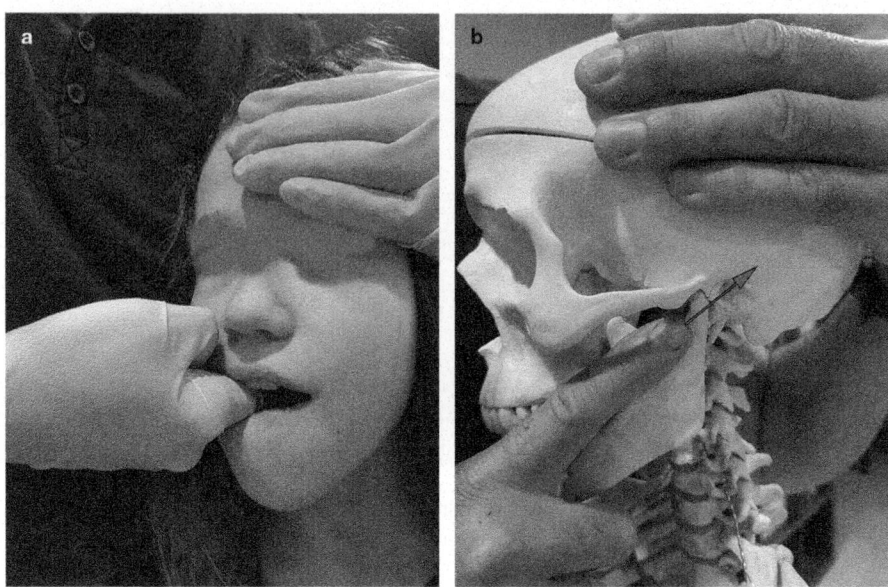

Fig. 7.13 Manipulation of the M. masseter is done with the fingertip laterally of the lower jaw in the pocket between the cheek and bone. The masseter is gently sprung backward

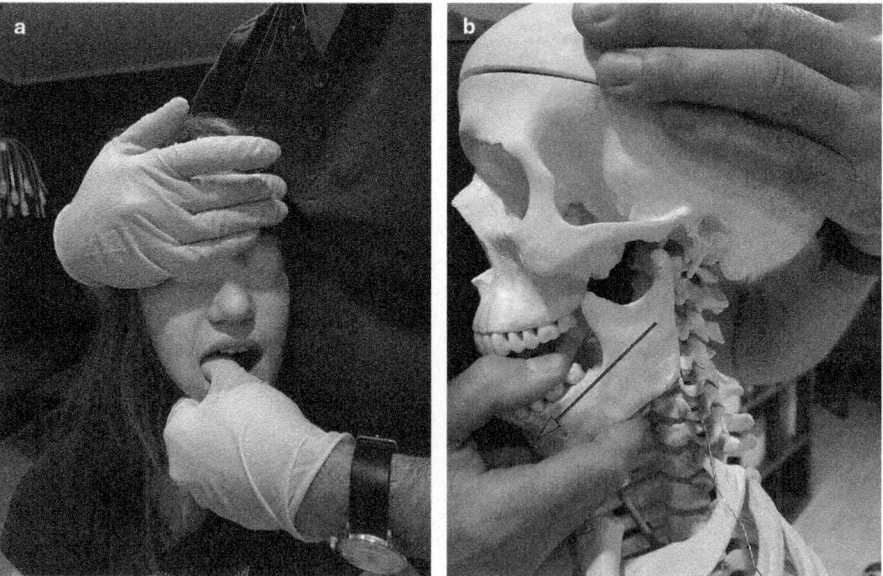

Fig. 7.14 Mobilization of the temporomandibular joint through resilient pulling movements forward and downward, pulling direction parallel to the row of teeth

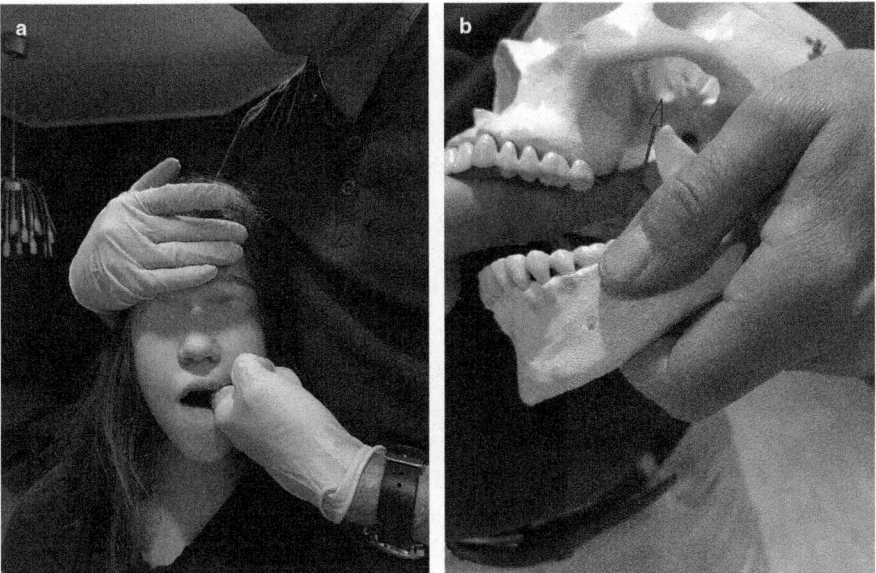

Fig. 7.15 The mobilization of the M. pterygopalatinus is done again with the fingertip of the index finger, which is placed behind the hard palate and the muscle is gently moved cranially

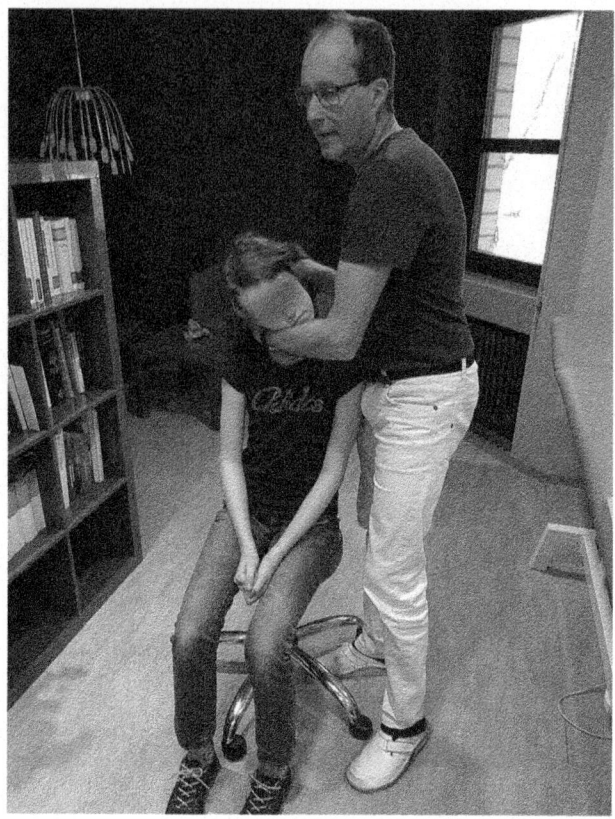

Fig. 7.16 Deblocking of the cervical segments. No force should be applied during all manipulations. Everything must be done gently; if the patient resists, wait until they relax

The Knot Model from a Physiotherapeutic Perspective— The KLINEA Concept

8

For over twenty years, I have been a physiotherapist. Like most of my colleagues, I have attended numerous further education courses during this time. When I have honest conversations with colleagues about the topic of "further education," we always come to the same conclusion: from each—often expensive—event, we picked out a few techniques that are useful in everyday work. Often, one could learn these "quintessences" of further education much faster and completely dispense with time-consuming ballast. Most teaching content and training trends lack coherent concepts in which the learned treatment techniques find structured explanations and lead to coherent treatment strategies. Ideally, a practical, pragmatic concept should consist of the essences of all these further education courses, without being artificially inflated and complicated. That is why I developed the KLINEA technique. The concept should primarily achieve the following:

- Ensuring a uniform treatment level from the career entrant to the experienced therapist in the team.
- Structuring the assessment as goal-oriented and efficient as the treatment, so that the idea of the treatment strategy is easily understood by everyone in the team and can still be comprehended after a long time.
- The resources of a prescribed prescription should be optimally used, and the patient should feel a positive change when leaving the practice.

By achieving these goals, not only is satisfaction created for the patient, but also for the prescribing doctor, the treating therapist, and ultimately, cost savings serve the general public.

In the following part of this book, the KLINEA concept is only briefly summarized in its approaches. So, there are hardly any detailed treatment strategies here. Rather, the functional thought pattern with which physiotherapists work should be presented. A detailed version of the KLINEA concept will be published soon in a separate book by Springer.

While doctors primarily work in the node area and treat acute complaints, the KLINEA concept also covers the functional chains (=fascial chains) in between, in addition to the node areas. These chains are often significantly involved in the complaints and must be treated as well.

The model assumes that all acute symptoms have their cause in nodes. If these are not treated promptly at the site, the body reacts with compensatory mechanisms that throw us off balance. This, in turn, leads to protective postures and disturbances in the functional chains.

In the KLINEA concept, the plumb line plays a crucial role. Often misinterpreted as "static" when it falls through the center of the body while standing, it should always be possible for the patient to comfortably bring themselves into the plumb line, as the least energy is expended in this position. However, it is already sufficient to briefly pass through the plumb line state to help the myofascial organ regenerate and detone, thus avoiding pathologies. Only when our organism experiences plumb line passages in its dynamics, which often only run through parts of the whole, does it remain overall in balance and free of blockages.

For example, if a tennis player's playing arm does not repeatedly reach the plumb line during the movement sequence in the game, i.e., does not balance the arm in the dynamics, they must expend more force, leading to poorer, more energy-consuming technique and, over time, to tension, myogeloses, and ultimately to overuse syndromes with tendinitis and insertion tendopathies.

The Assessment in KLINEA

9

Due to the general dynamics of our body, a static examination and therapy are not appropriate. Therefore, it is important to observe the patient even before entering the treatment room—when they do not yet expect to be "examined"—to watch them. In this way, before the actual examination, the following can be assessed: How does a patient sit in the waiting area, how do they get up, how do they walk, how do they undress?

From these impressions, initial conclusions can be drawn about the current posture and flexibility of the patient's musculoskeletal system. If the patient moves, for example, rather woodenly, it can be assumed that disturbances in the functional chains have persisted for a longer time. These important first observations are recorded to be able to refer to them for re-examination during the course of therapy.

As already described in the medical part of the book, KLINEA also works with the helpful node model, which is supplemented by the recording of force/tension vectors in between. Through this representation in the examination, the therapist saves time-consuming wordy descriptions, because vectors make three-dimensional axis deviations understandable. This type of representation is intuitively understood by all involved therapists. The vectors are illustrated by arrows, differentiating between disturbances within the individual nodes and the areas in between. In contrast to the medical view, in physiotherapy, the calotte, sacral, and foot nodes play a major role in the myofascial organ. If there is a disturbance in the foot node, this inevitably has consequences for the ascending functional chain and must be treated primarily. Disturbances in the calotte node provoke transmitted misinformation to caudal, so that the sacral node is another physiotherapeutic focus. Disturbances in the sacral node are particularly serious because this is where the body's center of gravity lies, which directly affects the individual plumb line posture.

9 The Author(s), under exclusive license to Springer-Verlag GmbH, DE, part of Springer Nature 2023
R. Eichinger and K. Klink, *Myofascial Pain and Dysfunction*,
https://doi.org/10.1007/978-3-662-68041-4_9

67

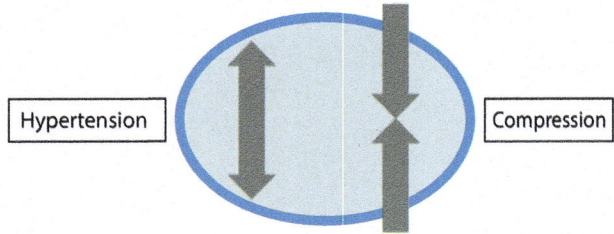

Fig. 9.1 Representation of a disturbance in the node in the examination

Each individual node can have a functional disorder on its own. This is subsequently referred to as "compression"and "hypertension"named. The compressed side can also be recognized as the "short side" in the examination, while the opposite node side shows hypertension. This is done using two arrows that meet at the tip (Fig. 9.1).

Since a compressed side always has a hypertension side opposite it, it is sufficient to mark the compressed side.

I would like to illustrate the model of compression and hypertension using a bow, where the compressed side corresponds to the tendon side, and the hypertension, or tension side, corresponds to the convex side of the bow. If the tension of the bowstring decreases, the bow wood relaxes equally. However, if you pull on the string, the tension of the bow increases immediately. Myofascial geloses can exist on both sides, but the pain predominantly occurs on the hypertension side. In a strongly kyphotic patient, this means that their pain usually occurs dorsally, in the area of the apex of the curvature, but this tension quickly subsides as soon as the ventral thorax finds relaxation. The therapy is therefore often carried out on the opposite side of the pain (Fig. 9.2).

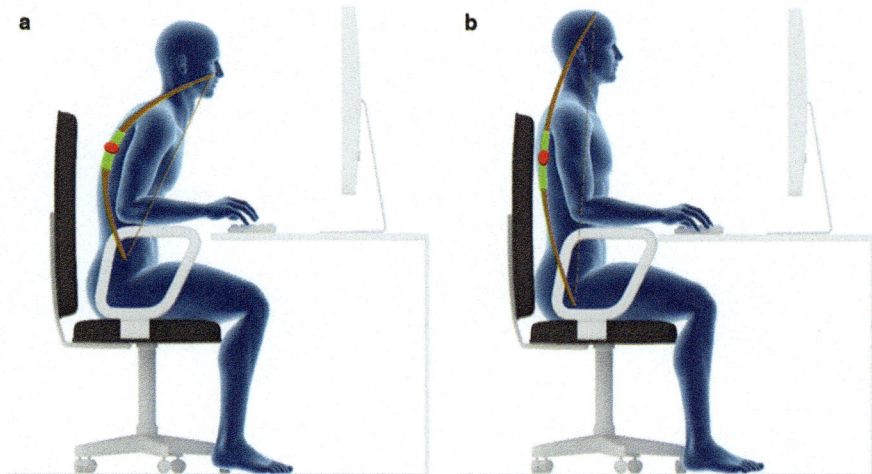

Fig. 9.2 Example office worker. While a kyphotic stress posture causes compression ventrally, the hypertension side comes under tension. Over time, the mobility of the ventral fascial chain decreases, and the patient can no longer comfortably reach their functional plumb line. Strengthening exercises for the dorsal trunk muscles also do not lead to lasting success here. Rather, the release of the ventral fascial chain by a therapist is indicated. Subsequent strengthening measures, which the patient should continue, complete the treatment

Pathophysiological Considerations from the Physiotherapist's Perspective

10

In physiotherapy, work is essentially done mechanically on and in the connective tissue. However, the question arises whether the mode of action of the therapy is actually purely mechanical. I do not believe so.

The myofascial organ is highly complex and also neurologically integrated into all body functions, so physiotherapy certainly does not work "only" mechanically.

All structures of our body, such as muscles, organs, nerves, blood vessels, etc., are enveloped in connective tissue. In order to be able to follow each of our everyday movements, these structures must be connected, but at the same time be able to glide smoothly against each other so as not to lose their function. This is done by means of fascia, which are kept slippery by their serous wetting. If the sliding ability of the fascia decreases, for example due to the natural aging process, poor posture, or lack of movement, geloses or adhesions form in the tissue.

The mode of action of mobilizing techniques in physiotherapy is therefore probably not exclusively, as is often assumed, due to the mobilization of a single fascial structure, but rather receptors are addressed by displacement techniques. These receptors probably stimulate the production of fluid in the serous membranes and thus improve the mobility of different fasciae against each other.

Mobilizing techniques on vertebral and rib joints also seem to cause neurological reactions, as the effect is immediately apparent in an improved displaceability of the myofascial system. Vegetative efferents are probably activated, which regulate the tissue tension of the myofascial organ.

The defined nodes in the diagnostic and therapeutic concept thus represent neurological key centers from which the intervening functional chains are influenced. These fascial chains are always treated in physiotherapy as well.

In our daily practice, it has proven useful to first have disorders in node areas medically clarified. For example, thyroid pathologies should be investigated if

R. Eichinger and K. Klink, *Myofascial Pain and Dysfunction*, https://doi.org/10.1007/978-3-662-68041-4_10

recurrent blockages occur in the cervical node. If physiotherapeutic measures on the lumbar spine remain unsuccessful, more detailed examinations in the small pelvis are urgently required. Therefore, close, trusting cooperation at eye level between doctors and physiotherapists and all other involved therapists is always absolutely necessary.

KLINEA Assessment

11

Contents

Before each diagnosis, a medical history is taken. Then follows the:

11.1 Visual Examination While Standing

The patient is dressed only in underwear and placed on two personal scales, with each foot on a scale. The displays of the scales face outward to make the result easy to read. The patient is now asked to stand comfortably and fixate on a point in front of them. Engaging the patient in a brief conversation helps them relax more quickly and find their individual relaxation posture.

In order to better recognize posture pathologies, several plumb lines are drawn: in the frontal plane between the center of the back of the head and the promontory on the sacrum, as well as on the legs from the ischial tuberosity to the center of the calcaneus (Fig. 11.1).

This creates references that facilitate the assessment of individual nodes. The focus is on evaluating each node for compression and hypertension in the various planes. Since each compression automatically has a hypertension opposite it, the therapist records only the compression side using two arrows that meet at the tip (Figs. 11.2 and 11.3).

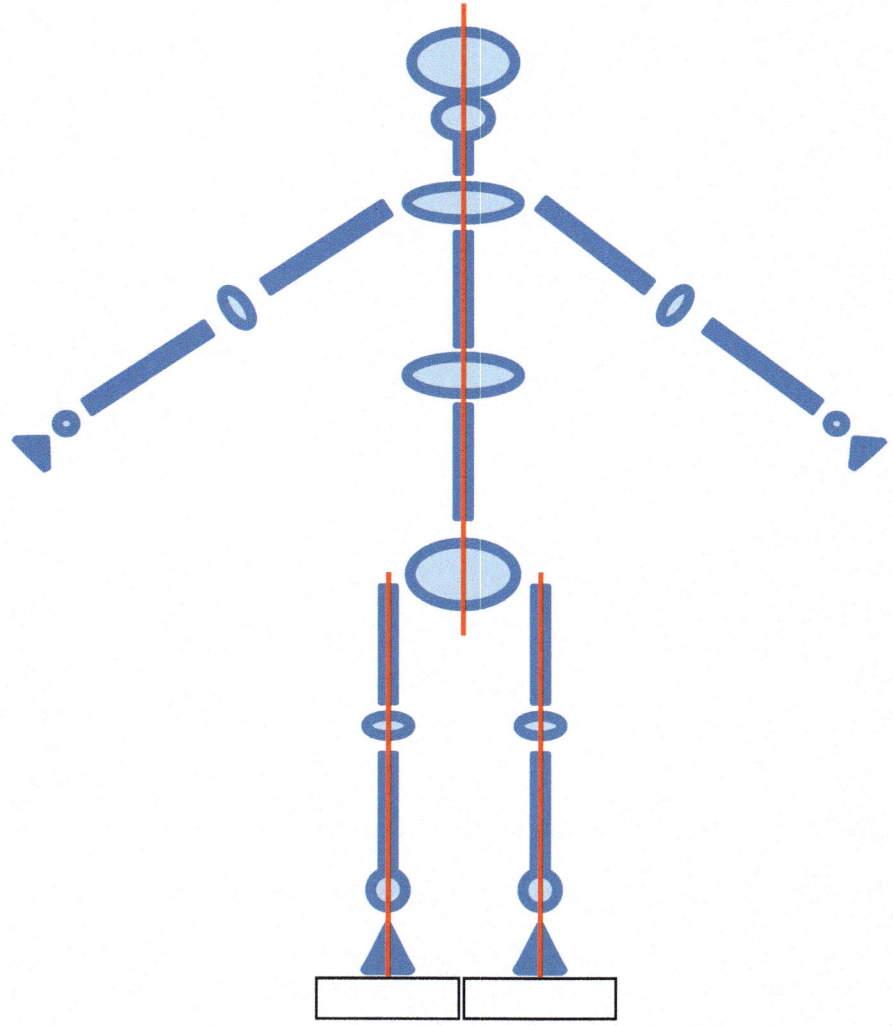

Fig. 11.1 Plumb lines of the frontal plane

In the KLINEA concept, in addition to the nodes, the internodal force vectors, which act via fascial chains, also play a central role. I find the evidence-based Tensegrity model very helpful here. The following are two excerpts from this model in graphics (Figs. 11.4 and 11.5).

If compressions are also found on the patient between the nodes, these are also marked with arrows.

For example, if a patient (Fig. 11.6) shows a steeper angle on the right side in the waist triangle, the compression is located on the right between the lower thoracic node and the sacral node.

a

Right foot node dorsal view **perpendicular**

b

Right foot node view ventrally laterally compressed

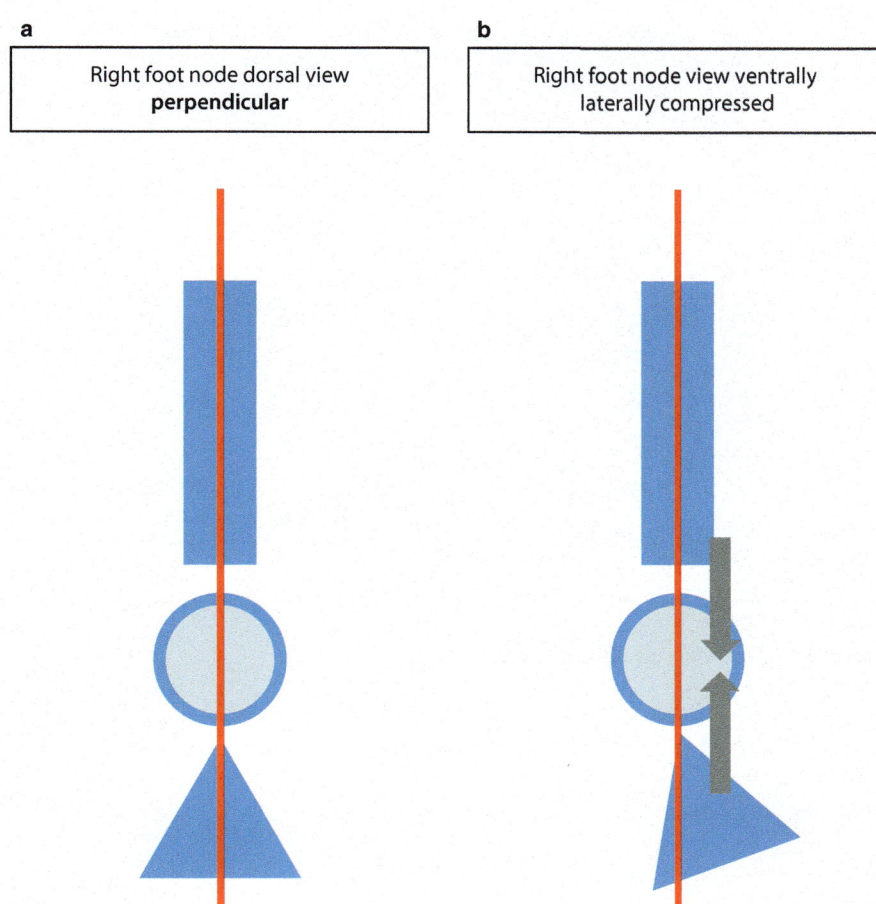

Fig. 11.2 Examination and documentation with compression and hypertension at the foot node

The evaluation from the lateral view is performed analogously (Fig. 11.7).

Subsequently, the weight difference between the two scales is examined. Initially, some patients sway because they often have a feeling of "giving in" on the scales. After a short time, most can stand still. Otherwise, we record an average from the fluctuation range and note this. We allow a tolerance range of approximately 3% of body weight as a difference. If there are higher side differences, a treatment-worthy finding is present, as the patient is too far out of plumb.

The scale test is also an excellent means of monitoring the course of therapy.

Chapter summary: Quick diagnostic tests for doctors and physiotherapists

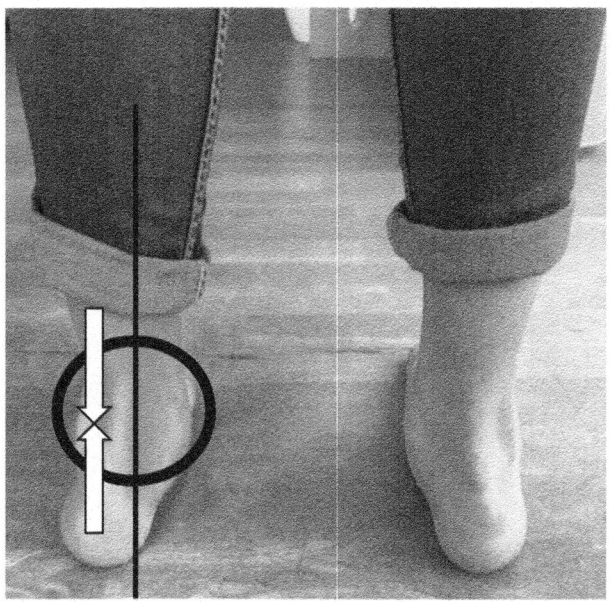

Fig. 11.3 Patient with laterally compressed foot node

11.2   Fast, Meaningful Practice Tests

In KLINEA treatment, three nodes play a special role:

- The calotte node as the highest point.
- The sacral node as the center of our functional plumb line.
- The foot node as the lowest point, carrying the entire body load.

Above all, these three nodes continuously provide information to the myofascial organ. For example, if the foot node has a compression, it sends incorrect information cranially with every step via the fascial leg chains, leading to imbalances in the subsequent nodes.

To determine which node requires treatment and how priorities should be set in the treatment, we use three important tests. The implementation in practice takes no more than three minutes.

11.2.1 Modified Derbolowsky Sign

For the detection of disturbances in the sacral and calvarial nodes

When referring to a leg length discrepancy (LLD) in the following, a functional leg length discrepancy is meant, which must not be confused with an anatomical one (e.g., after fractures). Blockages in the sacral node often make one leg appear

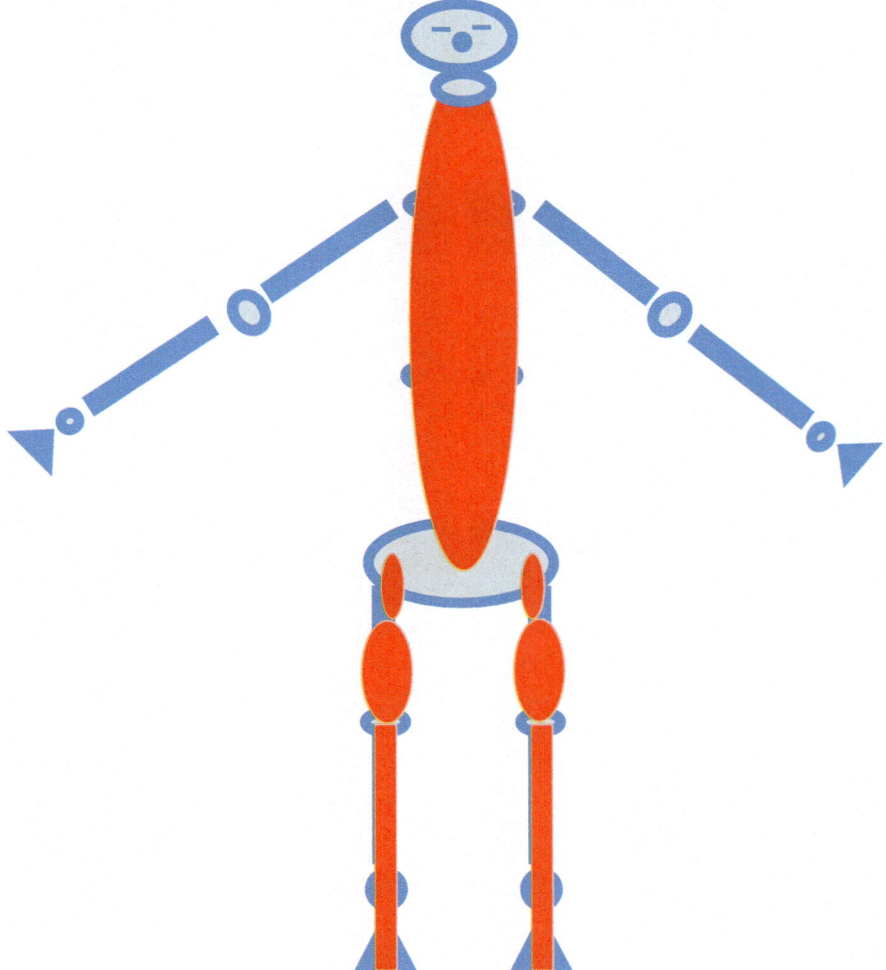

Fig. 11.4 Superficial ventral fascial functional chain according to the Tensegrity model

shorter because the pelvis pulls one leg upwards. The difference in length is purely functional.

The patient is in a supine position (SP). The therapist stands at the head end and first assesses the hip rotation using the patient's foot position; asymmetries are already an indication of blockages in the SN and should disappear during the course of therapy (Fig. 11.8).

Next, grasp the ankles from below and place the thumbs on the medial malleoli, then instruct the patient to pull both legs towards the chest to achieve a neutral position of the pelvis. Once the patient has laid their legs down again, the leg length is assessed at both medial malleoli. The patient is then asked to sit up and the leg length/difference is assessed again (Fig. 11.9).

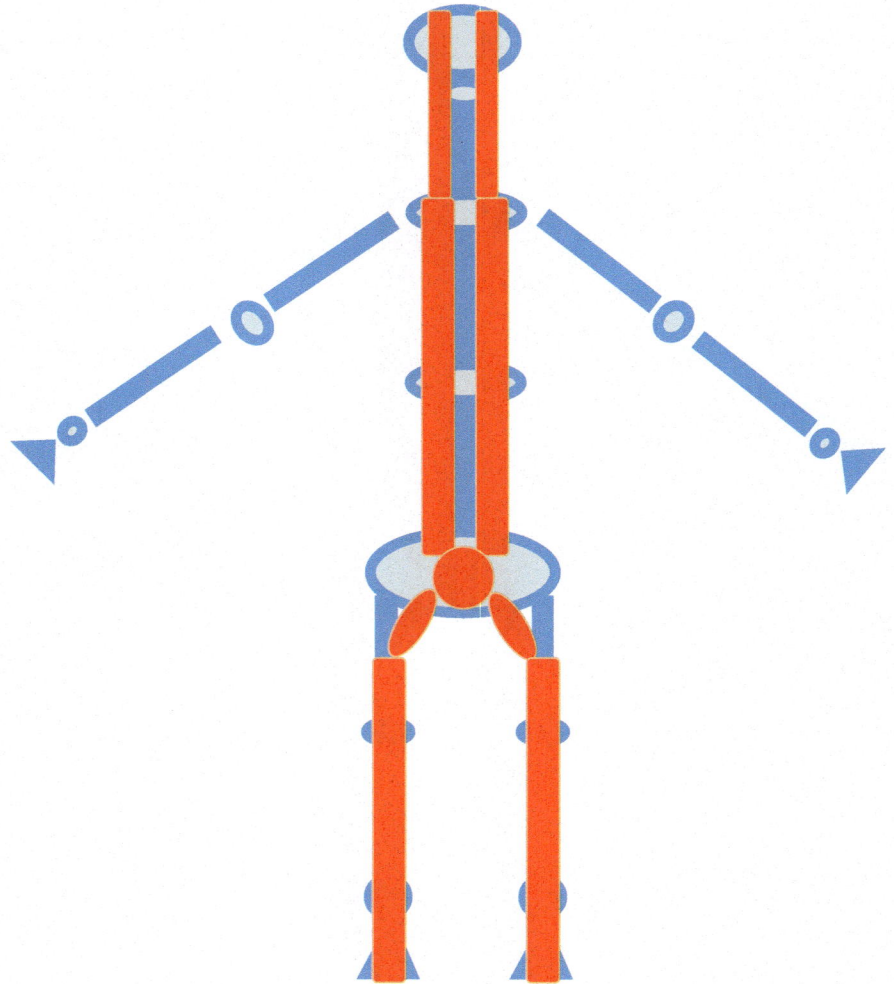

Fig. 11.5 Superficial dorsal fascial functional chain according to the Tensegrity model

The sitting up is repeated again. This time, the patient is instructed to clench their teeth during the movement to provoke the temporomandibular joint. The result of the leg lengths is noted afterward.

Assessment of the Test Functional leg length in supine position – sitting up

- Any change in the result (regardless of the change, it can also be that a previous leg length difference in the seat is suddenly balanced!) indicates a disturbance in the sacral node (e.g., a blockage of the sacrum or an SI joint).
- No change in the result makes involvement of the sacral node unlikely.

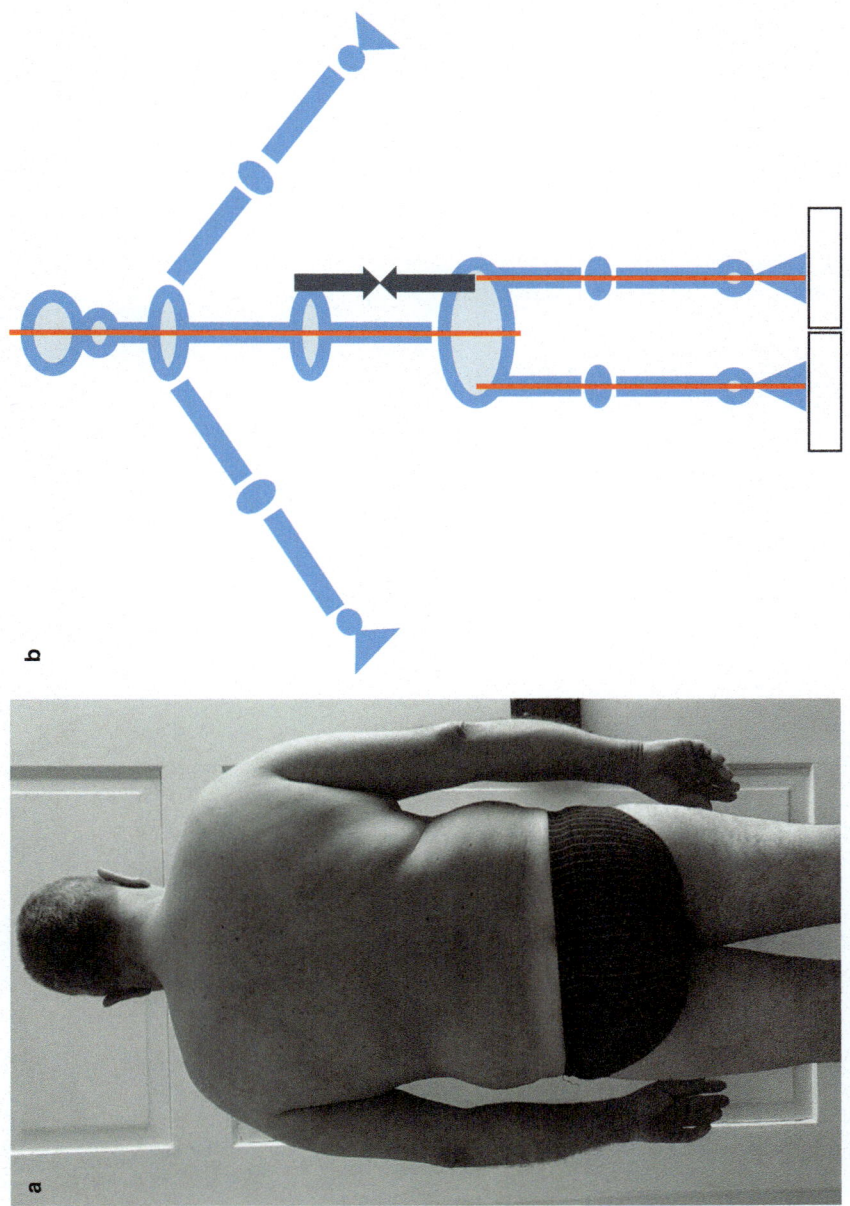

Fig. 11.6 Right-sided compression between the lower thoracic node and the sacral node, with the representation in the findings on the right

Fig. 11.7 Plumb line in the
lateral evaluation

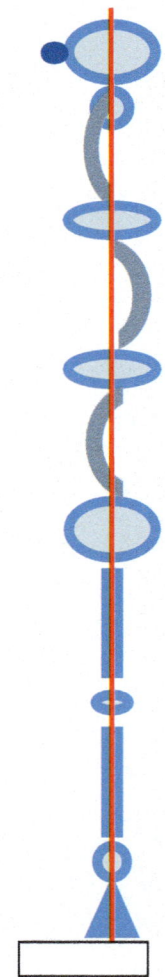

Functional leg length in supine position – sitting up with provocation of the temporomandibular joint

- Any change in the result indicates a disturbance in the calvarial or pharyngeal node.
- No change in the result makes a disturbance in the calvarial or pharyngeal node unlikely (Fig. 11.10).

11.2.2 Testing the Leg Chains

The patient lies in a supine position, with the arms positioned next to the body.

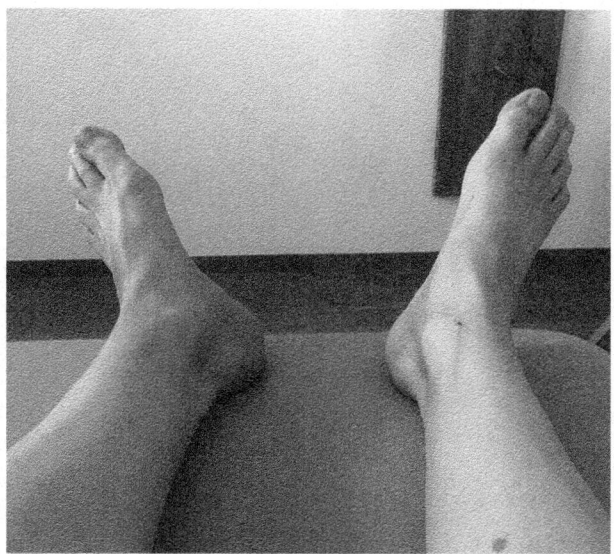

Fig. 11.8   Left leg rotated to the left via hip rotation

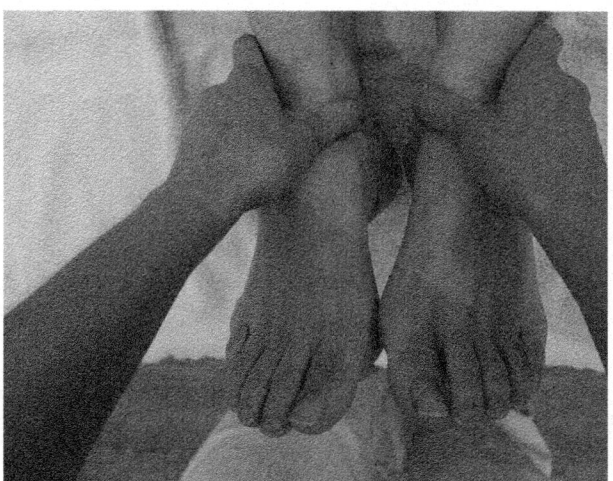

Fig. 11.9   Hand position during the modified Derbolowsky sign

Now, the therapist applies pressure to the upper ankle joints in the direction of plantar flexion and elastically rebounds at the endpoint to test flexibility in a side-by-side comparison. If one side reacts with a limited range of motion or does not rebound in the end position, this ventral leg chain is considered conspicuous (Fig. 11.11).

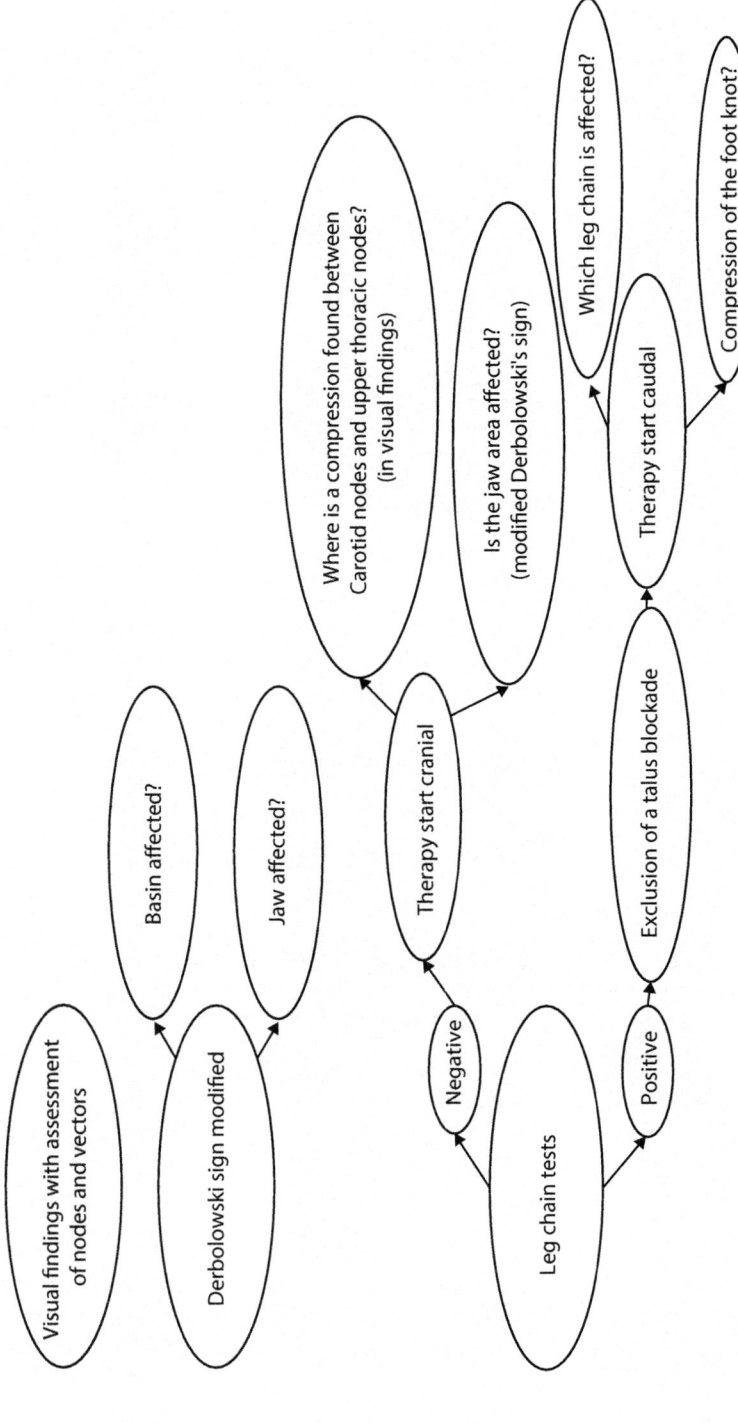

Fig. 11.10 Structured examination flowchart of the KLINEA technique

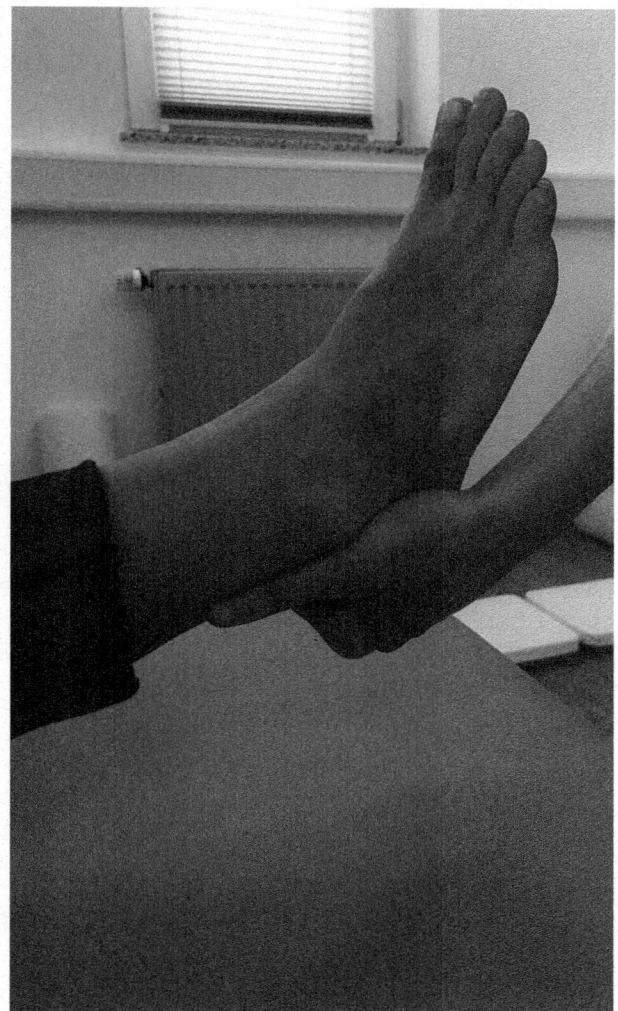

Fig. 11.11 Passive plantar flexion of the ankle joints during leg chain testing

The therapist proceeds in the same manner in dorsal extension. If a side difference is observed, the knee on the affected side is flexed about 30 degrees to deac-
tivate the dorsal fascial chain, and the test is repeated. If reduced dorsal extension
remains, we assume a talus blockage. This is resolved and tested again in knee
flexion and extension. If the patient still shows a unilateral limitation of dorsal
extension, increased tension in the dorsal leg chain is assumed.

To test the medial and lateral fascial chains of the legs, the starting position
remains the same. The therapist grasps both calcanei lumbrically (Fig. 11.12), lifts
them slightly off the surface, and moves the lower ankle joints in pronation and

Fig. 11.12 Lumbrical grip
for assessing leg chains

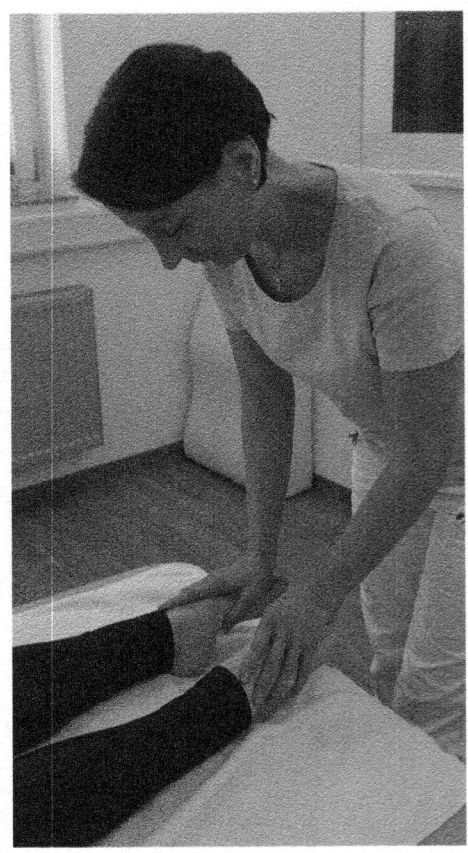

supination. In a side-by-side comparison, it becomes clear whether the medial or
lateral leg chain requires treatment (Fig. 11.12).

11.2.3 Toe Test

Another test for assessing leg chains is the toe test. Maximum traction is applied
to each toe. A blockage is present if traction does not allow separation of the toe
joint surfaces. If the joints are inconspicuous, they can be minimally pulled apart.
The test is also therapy, as the maneuver can individually unblock the toes, which
is often perceived as a bright cracking sound.

Results of the toe test:

Blockage of metatarsals IV and V: lateral leg chain is affected

Blockage of metatarsals I and II: medial leg chain is affected

Blockage of metatarsal III: dorsal or ventral leg chain is affected

KLINEA Therapy

12

Like all manual therapy treatment methods, the KLINEA technique is also a de-blocking, mobilizing procedure. With the fingertips, the proximal interphalangeal joint (PIP), and sometimes also with the ulnar edge of the forearm, fasciae are stretched, mobilized, and myogeloses are released. Those who treat a large number of patients "handmade" daily for years are at risk of developing arthritic changes in the finger joints due to this strain. The thumb saddle joints are particularly at risk. After 15 years in therapy, I also had problems with my finger joints. At times, I could no longer carry a full plate. Some treatments on patients could only be performed with pain. For this reason, I developed a treatment tool, the "Klimmi", which is mainly used for KLINEA treatment to protect the therapist. The Klimmi is made of medical silicone and is available in two different hardness levels. The material feels so natural on the patient's skin that the patient cannot distinguish it from the therapist's hand. The therapist's sensitivity is also fully preserved, unlike treatment aids made of wood or metal. The unbeatable advantage of the Klimmi, however, is that it does not have to be held like a pen by the fingers, but is simply placed in the dry palm of the therapist. The main load is thus distributed over the much more stable wrist during treatment. The pressure intensity is regulated by the use of body weight.

To make the Klimmi glide smoothly in the patient's tissue, it is necessary to use lotion or massage oil. The therapist's hand must remain completely dry (Fig. 12.1).

A decisive advantage of the KLINEA concept is the clear structuring that a therapist can follow. After performing the tests mentioned above, the therapist has gained an overview of the patient's myofascial organ and can proceed directly to treatment.

Procedure of the KLINEA therapy in brief:

The treatment begins either cranially at the carotid node descending to the sacral node or distally at the foot node ascending to the sacral node.

R. Eichinger and K. Klink, *Myofascial Pain and Dysfunction*,
https://doi.org/10.1007/978-3-662-68041-4_12

Fig. 12.1 Therapy aid
Klimmi in use

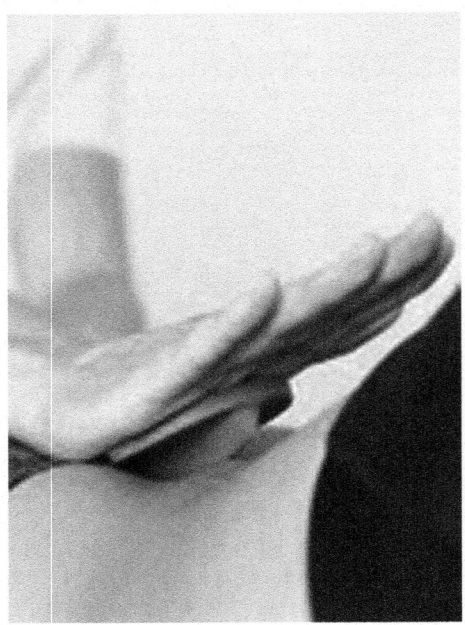

If involvement of the sacral node is confirmed, it is considered towards the end of the treatment, as it forms the center of our functional statics. Therefore, it should only be corrected when the distal structures can comfortably reach the functional plumb line.

The treatment in the nodes always begins on the compressed side, based on the visual findings. First, a mobility test of the tissue is performed in different directions and at different depths. The restricted direction is also the treatment direction. During this test, the therapist not only feels resistance in the tissue in the restricted direction but often also crepitations and nodular changes. These are adhesions or, in some literature, "tangling of the connective tissue" is mentioned, but ultimately these are variations of myogeloses.

The therapist is free to choose the mobilization technique. Sliding techniques with the fingertips, the PIPs, or using, for example, the Klimmi, or rolling and pinching grips are just a few examples of the possibilities.

Once the mobility has noticeably improved, the compression in the adjacent node or the affected internodal fascial chains is also treated.

A typical treatment course for an ascending problem, triggered by a medial compression of the foot node, would be, for example:

I.   Plantar fascia
II.   Releasing a talus blockage
III. Medial sliding bearing Achilles tendon
IV.   Transition Achilles tendon–Gastrocnemius

V. Ischiocrural fasciae
VI. Fascial structures around the buttocks, e.g., M. piriformis, M. obturatorius, etc.

If hardly any improvement can be achieved in one area, return to this node or vector at a later time. Often, better mobility can already be detected before another mobilization, as more distant adhered structures have often prevented improvement.

Shortly before the end of the therapy, the therapist addresses the sacral node.

This part of the treatment is deliberately described in more detail, as our focus is on the sacral node, more precisely in the promontory, which has a significant impact on the functional plumb line. If a disturbance of the sacral node was noticeable during the modified Derbolowsky sign, the question arises where the compression side was visible in the visual examination. A flexion of the hip joints in standing with a hyperlordosis of the lower lumbar spine is defined as ventral compression, for example. In this case, the ventrally running renal fascia is treated in the supine position after the direction of treatment has been determined using the mobility test. Relaxation of the renal fascia is indicated, among other things, by the fact that the distance between the patient's lumbar spine and the treatment couch becomes smaller (Fig. 12.2).

Now the correction of the pelvis follows in the prone position. Before that, a sliding test of the lumbar spine should be carried out urgently. If the lumbar spine is unable to extend, a sacrum mobilization in nutation provokes a sliding vertebra

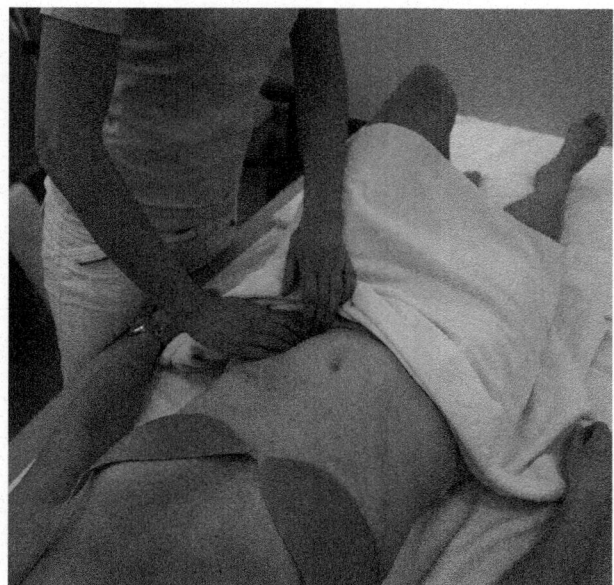

Fig. 12.2 Mobilization of the renal fascia in the area of the pelvic crest

L5/S1. In this test, pressure is applied to the spinous process L3-5 perpendicular to the lordosis curvature. If this slides gently into extension, the treatment can be continued. If a segment is unable to glide into extension, it is mobilized; otherwise, sacrum mobilization is contraindicated (Fig. 12.3).

Next, the ischiocrural test is performed in the prone position: the patient bends one leg at approximately 45 degrees. The therapist applies pressure to the calcaneus against knee flexion until the patient's strength level is reached and briefly increases the pressure. A well-functioning muscle should withstand this pressure. Cramp tendency is also interpreted as weakness. If the muscles react with weakness, the test is positive on this side. If the test is positive on both sides, it is a sacrum blockage. If only one-sided weakness is shown, an SI joint blockage is assumed. A brief impulse of the ilium in a mobilization direction, e.g., anterior, and an immediate re-test shows whether the treatment direction is correct. The same applies to the sacrum. In this way, all treatment directions of the pelvis can be quickly and reliably tested.

Fig. 12.3 Sliding test of the lumbar spine in extension

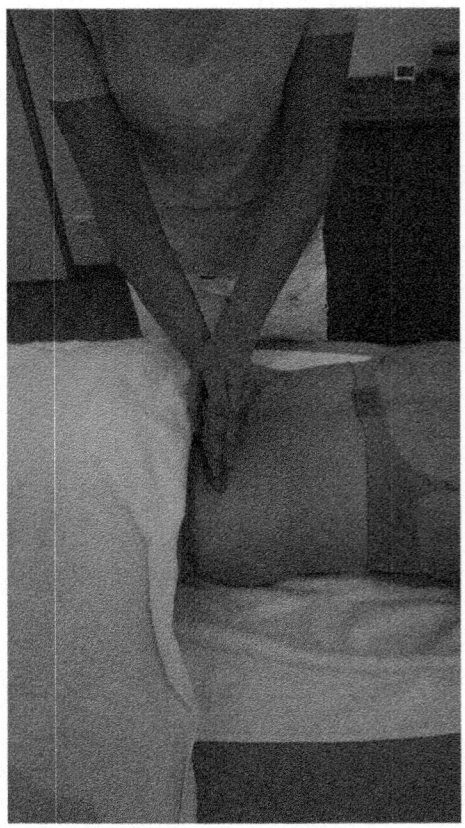

While the modified Derbolowsky-test shows, **whether** *the pelvis has a dysfunction, the ischiocrural test shows,* **where** *the blockage is located and in* **which direction it needs to be regulated** .

After the appropriate mobilization of the sacrum and/or SI joint, the result is checked with the ischiocrural test. Only when both leg flexors can withstand pressure and repressure without any problems is the pelvis free of blockages.

After a completed treatment unit, all tests are performed again. In the re-examination immediately following the first treatment, they should all be significantly improved, ideally even inconspicuous.

The weight distribution between right and left does not necessarily have to be balanced after a treatment. Instead, tension regulation creates an opportunity for the body to rediscover its functional plumb line in the various planes.

If a region of the patient was particularly noticeable during the treatment (by "noticeable" I mean an accumulation of myogeloses), self-mobilization is given to the patient as homework. This is where the therapist's creativity is needed. From experience, the guided use of softer, structure-permeated fascia rollers is useful, and a cork can also be used to mobilize the plantar fascia. For point-specific self-treatments, e.g., on the legs, the Klimmi has proven to be a suitable aid. Regular stretching exercises during seated activities and sufficient exercise as a balance in leisure time should be passed on by therapists as useful tips rather once too often. As with all structures in the body, the same applies to the myofascial organ: "use it or lose it."

Patient Example

13

Contents

13.1 Medical History

28-year-old female patient, varied work, hobbies: ballroom dancing, jogging, and (rather rarely) climbing. Status post tonsillectomy and appendectomy in childhood. The appendectomy was preceded by a highly acute appendicitis. The patient was unable to participate in sports for 8 months.

Complaints:

- Pain in the right Achilles tendon for 9 months, even at rest, pain radiating along the gastrocnemius to the popliteal fossa during dancing
- Feeling of instability in the left knee joint while dancing
- Pain in the right sacroiliac joint for 4 years
- Nonspecific gastrointestinal complaints (medically evaluated, diagnosis: irritable bowel syndrome) for 4 years
- Pain and tension in the right occiput, radiating into the neck for 2 years

Half a year ago, the patient consulted an orthopedist to have her Achilles tendon treated. After 3 cortisone injections, the patient discontinued the therapy as no improvement was noticeable. Local physiotherapeutic techniques also remained unsuccessful at that time.

Four months ago, the patient presented to Dr. Eichinger. After chirotherapy on the lumbar spine/pelvis and cervical spine, the pain shifted from the sacroiliac joint to the right groin area when the abdominal muscles were activated. The remaining complaints improved only slightly. After an injection of the appendix scar with bupivacaine and another chirotherapy, the complaints in the Achilles tendon and groin improved by 40%, while the remaining complaints remained almost unchanged. The patient then presented to our practice for KLINEA treatment.

13.2   Visual Findings

Balance test, a side difference of approximately 14% of body weight is shown (Figs. 13.1, 13.2, 13.3 and 13.4)

13.3   Quick Tests

After the visual findings, the patient moved into a supine position. Here, a significant external rotation of the right hip joint was observed.

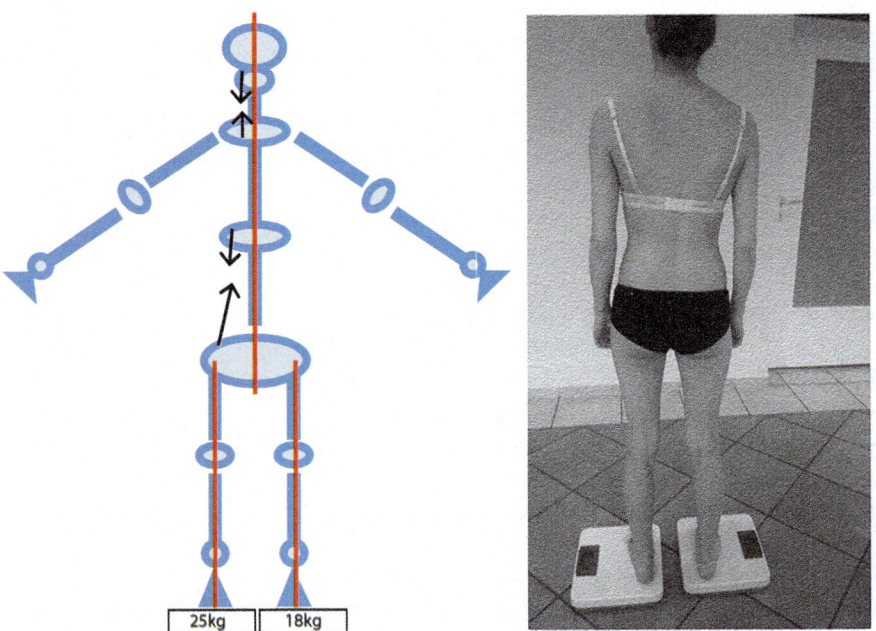

25kg   18kg

Fig. 13.1 Dorsal visual findings with documentation in the node model: Compression between pharyngeal node and upper thoracic node on the left, compression between lower thoracic node and sacral node on the left, and lateral compression of the right foot node. The weight difference is documented as a reference

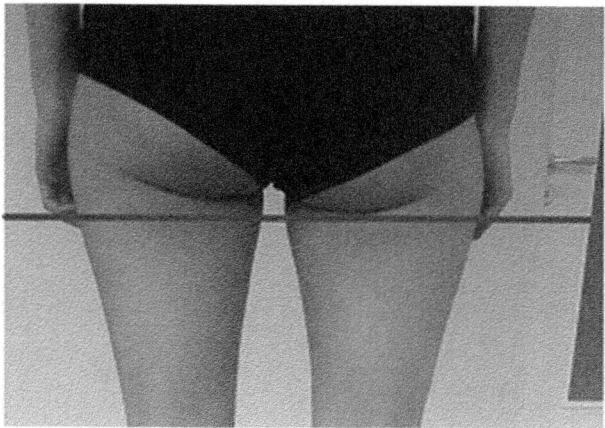

Fig. 13.2 The right gluteal fold is significantly lower than the left

The modified Derbolowsky test clearly indicated a disturbance in the sacral node and calotte node.

The leg chain test revealed involvement of the ventral and lateral leg chain right > left. Even releasing the talus blockage on the right did not yield an improved result. The toe test confirmed this. The severely restricted mobility of the leg fascia justifies the suspicion of ascending symptoms, which is why the therapy begins caudally, but later focuses on the sacral node.

13.4 Therapy

- Fascia release of the
  - ventral and lateral leg chains up to the sacral node.
  - Scalp up to the suboccipital musculature.
  - ventral thoracic fascia with diaphragm.
  - left lateral thoracic fascia in the area of the M. quadratus lumborum.
- Manual therapeutic mobilization of the cervicothoracic and thoracolumbar transition in extension. If the body has the possibility to straighten up better through a ventral fascia release, the cervicothoracic and thoracolumbar transition must also be able to allow this newly gained mobility.

Afterwards, the intermediate test on the scales showed only a difference of 4 kg.

- Due to the anamnesis, the appendix scar was manually tested for mobility. The cranio-medial direction was restricted in both superficial and deep layers and was treated as well.

Fig. 13.3 Lateral visual findings with documentation in the node model. Dorsal compression between calotte node and upper pharyngeal node, ventral compression between upper and lower thoracic nodes, ventral compression in the lower thoracic node, dorsal compression in the sacral node, and ventral compression in the knee node

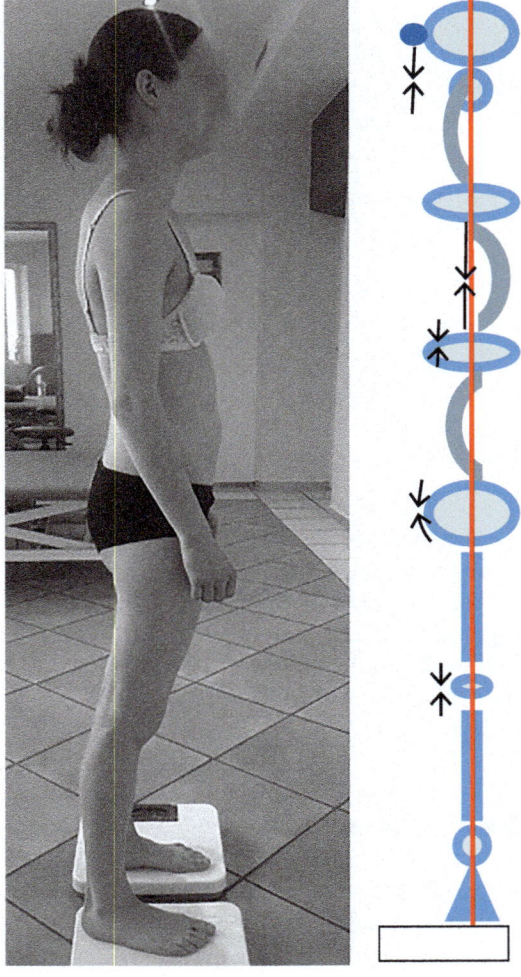

- In the ischiocrural test, a significant weakness was evident on both sides. After treatment of the sacrum in nutation, only the right side showed noticeable weakness. After the right SIJ was mobilized in the anterior direction, the ischiocrural test was negative on both sides.

13.5   Findings

- Ischiocrural test bilaterally: negative (both leg flexors showed no more weakness)
- Modified Derbolowsky sign: negative. (Leg length difference was balanced with and without jaw provocation)

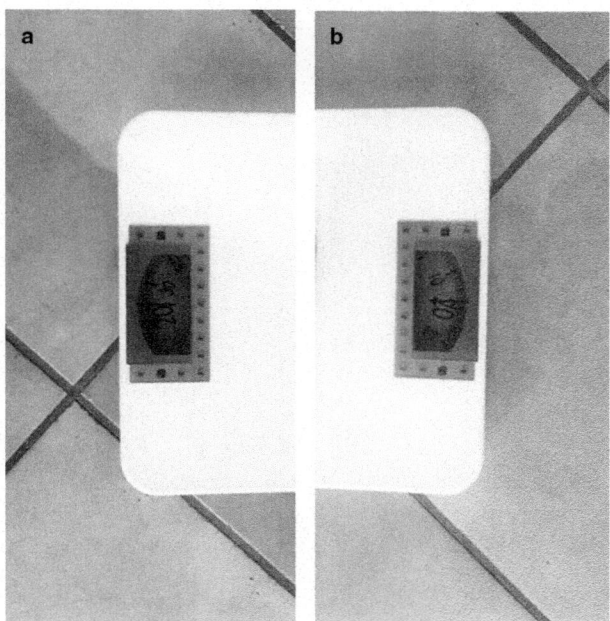

Fig. 13.4 The scales show a weight difference of 7 kg, with the left side being more loaded

- Leg chain test: negative (both ankle joints showed no more restrictions in any direction) (Figs. 13.5, 13.6 and 13.7)

After 3 weeks, we contacted the patient as agreed, and she reported that after the treatment, no groin pain and no neck pain had occurred, the Achilles tendon complaints were only noticeable during movement, and the pain had disappeared at rest. The gastrointestinal symptoms were reduced by only about 30% according to the patient.

After another 3 weeks, the patient informed me again about the current state of her health. The gastrointestinal symptoms remained the same. For two weeks, the pain in her Achilles tendon had disappeared, which prompted her to attempt a first running training. After the run, a slight "whimpering" in the Achilles tendon was noticeable, which lasted for 3 hours. She also mentioned that her running style felt "smoother." Only now did she report a previous asymmetry while jogging, which had disappeared after the treatment. Dancing would continue for her and her partner in the next season.

Fig. 13.5 The compressions
in the nodes and vectors were
almost completely resolved

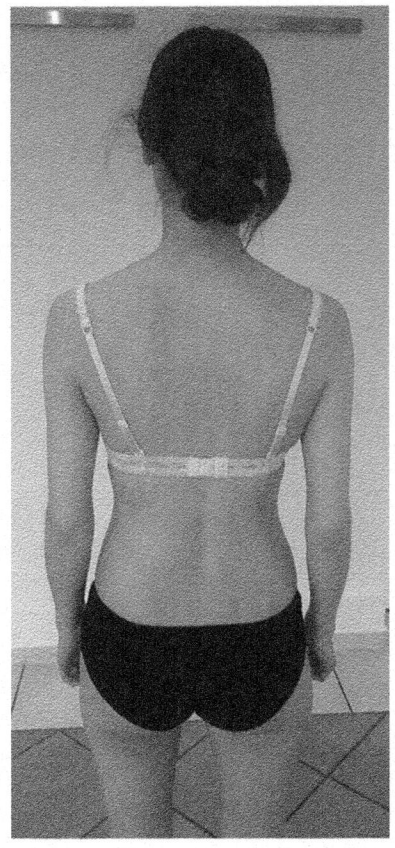

Fig. 13.6 The gluteal fold is
almost back in line

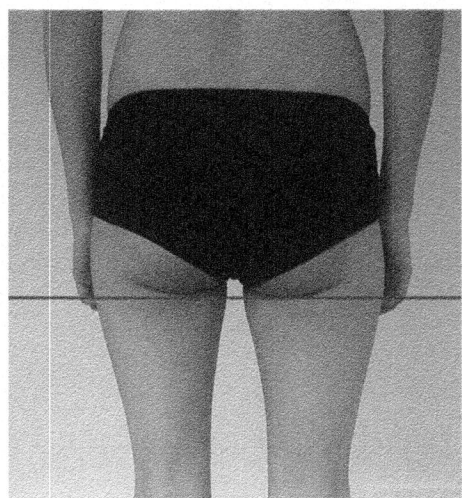

Fig. 13.7 The scales were completely balanced at the end of the treatment. The patient was given the task of regularly mobilizing the scar and incorporating exercises for upright posture into her daily routine

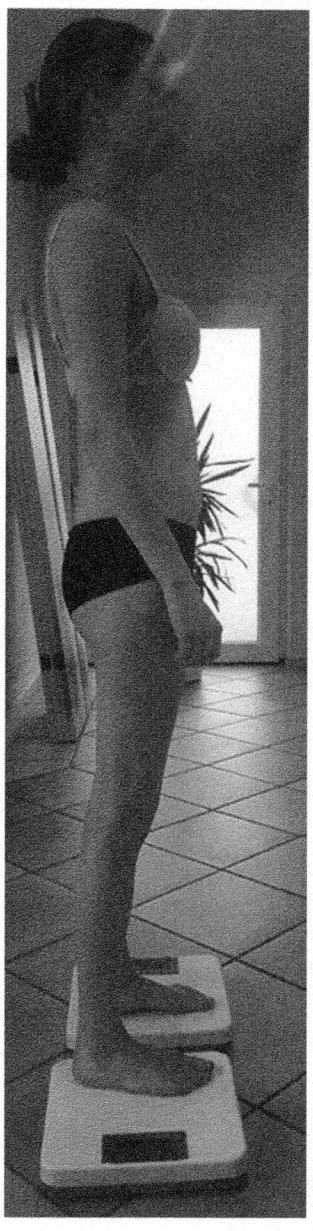

Afterword

We hope that this book has contributed a little to the understanding and treatment of myogeloses. The frequency of diseases of the myofascial organ should necessarily become an important topic in the education of doctors and physiotherapists. We are confident that we will still experience these developments.

Note

Many diagnostic and therapeutic processes are much easier to understand in demonstration videos. You can find these on our website at www.myofaszial.eu.

The manufacturer's authorised representative in the EU is Springer
Nature Customer Service Centre GmbH, Europaplatz 3, 69115 Heidelberg,
Germany. If you have any concerns regarding our products, please
contact ProductSafety@springernature.com

Printed and bound by CPI Group (UK) Ltd, Croydon, CR0 4YY
24/04/2026
02096356-0001